Psychology of Emotions, Motivations and Actions

Emotional First Aid on the Internet

Theory and Research

Psychology of Emotions, Motivations and Actions

Additional books in this series can be found on Nova's website under the Series tab.

Additional e-books in this series can be found on Nova's website under the e-book tab.

PSYCHOLOGY OF EMOTIONS, MOTIVATIONS AND ACTIONS

EMOTIONAL FIRST AID ON THE INTERNET

THEORY AND RESEARCH

ITZHAK GILAT
HANNA EZER
AND
RACHEL SAGEE

nova publishers
New York

Library of Congress Cataloging-in-Publication Data

Emotional first aid on the Internet: theory and research / editors, Itzhak Gilat, Hanna Ezer and Rachel Sagee.
pages cm. -- (Psychology of emotions, motivations and actions)
Includes bibliographical references and index.
ISBN 978-1-62948-568-3 (hardcover)
1. Hotlines (Counseling) 2. Internet--Social aspects. 3. Mental health services. 4. Mental health counseling. I. Gilat, Itzhak.
RC480.6.E465 2014
362.2'04251--dc23

2014036529

Published by Nova Science Publishers, Inc. † New York

CONTENTS

PREFACE

Marshall McLuhan coined the famous expression, "The medium is the message" (1964), long before communication went online. This expression reflects the idea that the environment in which communication occurs is not merely a passive channel for transmitting messages, but can also affect the nature of communication with regard to both its process and outcome. No medium of communication has provided such dramatic evidence of this idea as the online environment.

One of the domains of communication that was substantially affected by the Internet is psychotherapy along with other types of emotional assistance. Both clinical experience and research evidence have revealed that some features of the online environment may not only enhance people's willingness to seek assistance but also increase its efficacy (Barak, 2007; Lester, 2008-2009; Skinner & Zack, 2004; Suler, 2004). More specifically, the option to remain anonymous reduces the barriers of stigma and shame; the fact that assistance is easily available is particularly valuable to individuals in crisis who are in need of immediate relief; the use of written texts for communication promotes openness and self-disclosure; and the diverse modes of communication (e.g., synchronous, asynchronous, individual, group) can meet the needs of a variety of populations.

One of the earliest contexts of Internet-based psychological assistance was emotional first aid. Although individuals who are experiencing crisis require immediate support, many of them eschew seeking formal professional assistance due to practical limitations such as cost, low rate of accessibility to mental health agencies, or psychological barriers such as shame and the need for self-reliance (Garland & Zigler, 1994; Gilat, Ezer & Sagee, 2011). Volunteer-based telephone hotlines seem to be an appropriate source of assistance for such individuals. Indeed, the history of the mental health services shows that hotlines have proliferated since their first appearance in the mental health arena in the 1960s, and have become a unique and valuable source of crisis intervention, suicide prevention, and other types of emotional first aid.

Online emotional first-aid services can be described as a natural extension of volunteer-based telephone hotlines. The online environment not only shares the advantages of the telephone, which enhance emotional assistance, but also possesses additional features that can increase the efficacy of such assistance. It is not surprising that emotional first aid was offered on the Internet soon after communication went online (Wilson & Lester, 2002). This service began by responding to individuals who sought assistance via email, and expanded to other online applications such as the personal chat and online support groups.

There is a dearth of empirical evidence pertaining to the emotional first aid provided by trained volunteers on the Internet. Most of the existing evidence is based on clinical experience and field projects rather than on systematic studies. The present book is an attempt to remedy the lack of research evidence by presenting the findings of studies examining the process and the content of emotional first aid on the Internet, as well as theoretical perspectives regarding various aspects of this particular mental health service. The studies were conducted within the context of ERAN, The Israeli Association for Emotional First Aid.

The first chapter of the book presents an overview of volunteer-based emotional first-aid services. Emotional first aid via the Internet developed as an extension of the telephone helpline immediately after communication went online. The chapter focuses on the telephonic roots of the Internet service, presenting the historical background of the telephone helpline, describing its advantages and limitations, and reporting empirical findings as regards its effectiveness.

The second chapter shifts the focus of attention to the online environment and portrays the characteristics of the types of online environment that enhance psychological assistance. Both the willingness to receive emotional assistance and the process of rendering assistance are significantly affected by the specific features of the Internet. The chapter describes these features and presents empirical evidence of the increasing popularity of the Internet as a context for offering emotional support.

The purpose of the third chapter is to create a profile of the individuals who seek emotional first aid from trained volunteers on the Internet. Two components of the profile are presented: the characteristics of the individuals who choose to seek help in this unique environment, and the characteristics of the problem domains that these individuals present to the volunteers. The profile is based on a survey of 600 naturally-occurring online interactions retrieved from the ERAN database –200 interactions in each of the three channels that ERAN offers to the Israeli public, namely, personal chat, email, and an online support group. A comparison is drawn among the three channels with regard to both the characteristics of the help-seekers and the problem domains presented by them.

The fourth chapter foregrounds the personal chat and explores its value as a source of emotional assistance for individuals who are unwilling to seek help from face-to-face sources. Help-seekers suffering from Anorexia Nervosa (AN) and those experiencing trauma following sexual assault were chosen to serve as the research participants in view of the difficulty involved in seeking face-to-face emotional help – a difficulty that is inherent in both disorders. The findings are based on the in-depth, qualitative analysis of twelve transcripts of conversations between female help-seekers and trained volunteers that took place via the personal chat. The analyses reveal the unique contribution of the personal chat in situations in which face-to-face assistance elicits only limited improvement.

The fifth chapter focuses on one of the earliest online applications used for rendering emotional first aid, namely, email. The chapter expounds the advantages and limitations of email as a mode of online assistance. It further presents empirical evidence regarding three aspects of the interaction between individuals who seek emotional first aid via email and ERAN's volunteers: (1) the domains of the problems presented by the help-seekers; (2) the type of assistance the help-seekers expect to receive; and (3) the response strategies employed by the volunteers in order to provide assistance. Finally, the advantages of email, the type of assistance, and the response strategies are exemplified in a case study of an interaction between a troubled adolescent and a trained volunteer.

Online support groups – the virtual version of face-to-face support groups – constitute the focal point of the sixth chapter. The latter presents the theoretical background of the three components of the phenomenon: social support, therapeutic value of group processes, and online environment. Both the advantages and limitations of online support groups are described. Empirical evidence pertaining to the helpfulness of these groups is presented, and the effect of such a group moderated by trained volunteers is illustrated by means of an analysis of an entire thread retrieved from the online support group operated by the ERAN.

The seventh chapter presents two studies in order to address the issue of the helpfulness of the emotional first aid. The first study examined the perceptions of 118 individuals who responded to a questionnaire that examined their level of satisfaction with an interaction with a volunteer via the personal chat. The second study was based on a qualitative analysis of transcripts of chats that were defined as helpful in accordance with predetermined criteria. The analysis shed light on the components that characterize helpful interactions and expound the implications for practice and training.

The limitations, risks, and ethical dilemmas associated with providing emotional first aid on the Internet are presented and discussed in the eighth chapter. First, the limitations and risks that are common to professional therapy and emotional first aid are put forward: dependence on technology, faking, lack of non-verbal cues, and encouragement of dangerous behaviors such as suicide and eating disorders. Subsequently, ethical dilemmas that are specific to the context of volunteer-based emotional first aid are described and discussed: dealing with recurrent help-seekers as well as with suicidal individuals who contact a service that offers assistance, but refuse to cooperate with its efforts to help them deal with their crises.

In view of the enormous discrepancy between the needs of individuals worldwide for mental health assistance on the one hand and the availability of traditional formal sources on the other, it is justifiable to expand the types of mental health assistance offered to the population (Kazdin & Blasé, 2011). Volunteer-based emotional first aid is most appropriate for this purpose. We hope that this book will stimulate interest in this unique and valuable mode of mental assistance, enhance its application, and encourage its investigation.

We would like to thank the Israel Internet Association [ISOC-IL] for supporting the research with a grant.

Itzhak Gilat, Hanna Ezer and Rachel Sagee
Levinsky College of Education
Tel Aviv, Israel

Corresponding Author
Prof. Itzhak Gilat
Levinsky College of Education
15 Percitz Street Tel-Aviv, Israel
Tel: 972-3-6902422
972- 52 -631682
E-mail: gilati@netvision.net.il

Chapter 1

EMOTIONAL FIRST AID: AN OVERVIEW

ABSTRACT

Emotional first aid on the Internet developed as an expansion of the volunteer-based telephone helpline as soon as communication went online. The theoretical concept and the practical models of the online service were adopted from the telephone helpline. The present chapter focuses on the telephonic roots of the Internet service.

Volunteer-based emotional first aid via the telephone (helpline) was developed in the late 1950s for the specific aim of suicide prevention. Applying the features of telephone communication (particularly client anonymity and a high degree of availability) and exploiting the advantages of trained volunteers for rendering emotional assistance, it became a unique and valuable source of assistance for a wide spectrum of problem domains, providing immediate assistance to millions worldwide. This chapter presents the historical background of the telephone helpline, describes its advantages and limitations, and reports empirical findings regarding its effectiveness.

INTRODUCTION

The following description was written by an Israeli hotline service (ERAN) volunteer who participated in a study focusing on the perceived effectiveness of interactions with callers to the hotlines. The volunteers were requested to recall a particularly effective call and transcribe it in detail (Gilat & Rosenau, 2011). The description was written by a female volunteer who received the call the day after a major terrorist attack that was perpetrated in the center of TelAviv during the second intifada.

> "The caller sounded extremely agitated. He chose his words very carefully. He never thought that he would call ERAN for help. He always advised others to get help from ERAN and there he was, in their situation. I carefully asked him what had happened. He told me that the previous dayhe was summoned to come immediately to a location where a terrorist attack had occurred. They called him since he had been working as a policeman in the emergency forces for about thirty years. He spent three hours there, doing the necessary tasks, working like a robot. Since that event, he has been unable to sleep; he keeps seeing the scenes and hearing the sounds of the event. He knows that everything is in his head, but it seems so realistic to him that he feels as if he is losing his mind. He said that he does not understand what is happening to him. He had never reacted so emotionally. People always counted on him, and now he wasn't managing to stay in control. The man burst into tears. It was the first time that he had cried. Nobody had ever seen him broken. He did not understand how he had collapsed. He wanted to know what was happening to him.
>
> I told him that his feelings were understandable and legitimate. I talked to him about the difficulty involved in managing such events over and over again. People break down because of a single event of this kind, while he had experienced dozens of them over the years. I suggested that he view his reaction not as a sign of weakness but rather as an indication of his humanity. This vulnerability proved that he is a human being. Everyone has a threshold beyond which they cannot tolerate pain. The glass is full and additional emotions overflow. I began to talk to him gently about the need to get immediate assistance. I told him that if the help is given soon after the traumatic event, it would be more effective. He replied that he had already visited a general practitioner who suggested that he see a psychiatrist. He had to wait four days for the appointment with the psychiatrist and he felt that he needed to talk to someone – anonymously. We continued to talk about seeking help in times of distress. I used the image of a tall tree that bends in a strong wind and straightens when the wind stops. He was very grateful that I was there to listen to him. I told him that I would extend my shift by an hour, and invited him to call me if he needed to do so. He asked me not to extend it and promised to take care of himself. 'This tree will bend temporarily and then straighten again."

The concluding section of the volunteer's response, in which she was requested to reflect upon her own experience regarding this conversation, illustrates the unique value of the telephone helpline as a means of providing emotional assistance.

> "I reconstructed the conversation in my head and came to the conclusion that the telephone encounter between me and the caller was actually a crisis intervention, as I had read in the professional literature and as I had learned in my training before beginning my shifts. Crisis is a powerful storm that disrupts the routine of normal people and engenders the need to get help from external sources. In many cases, people who experience crisis do not seek professional, face-to-face help because it is too threatening. The opportunity to talk on the phone, anonymously, enables them to receive the assistance they need so much. In many cases, the positive experience with the telephone conversation increases their willingness to proceed with the professional assistance that is necessary to help them return to normality, and even bolsters their inner strength."

The type of assistance chosen by the policeman, namely, the telephone conversation with the volunteer, suited his emotional needs while experiencing acute anxiety. He felt an immediate need to share his feelings in a supportive environment, where, as a result of his lack of experience in receiving psychological assistance, he felt emotionally safe to disclose his feelings anonymously. In addition, the person who responded to him was not a professional, but rather a trained volunteer who, thanks to her training, possessed the relevant knowledge about crisis.

The above-mentioned characteristics of the telephone helpline contributed to its popularity as a unique source of psychological assistance all over the world. In the following sections, we present the historical background of this service, its advantages and limitations, and empirical evidence pertaining to its effectiveness.

Historical Background

The use of the telephone for purposes of suicide prevention originated in 1906 when the Salvation Army, motivated by religious principles, founded the "Anti-Suicide Bureau" in London. That same year, The National Save-a-Life League established a similar service in New York (Trowell, 1979). About five decades later, a major development in the history of telephonic mental health assistance occurred in Britain and the USA with the establishment of the volunteer-based telephone helpline. The British and American services were inspired by different philosophies: the British organization, called "The Samaritans", was guided by religious values, while the American hotlines applied innovative conceptions in the fields of community psychology and mental health. However, on both sides of the ocean, the new mental health services shared the same objective and professional characteristics.

While the British vicar, Chad Vara, did not have any formal education in mental health, his experience in the community taught him that individuals who experience acute emotional distress simply wanted someone who would listen to them, in confidence, with acceptance and compassion; this willingness to listen could influence their decision either to commit suicide or to go on living. A critical event that triggered the establishment of the Samaritans was funeral of a 13-year-old girl who had committed suicide following the onset of her menstrual cycle. She had not had anyone to turn to, and her fear and guilt had driven her to kill herself (http://www.samaritans.org/).

The first emergency telephone service in the USA was inaugurated in Los Angeles in 1958 "for the evaluation, referral, treatment, follow-up and overall prevention of suicide behavior" and was followed by the establishment of hundreds of such centers in the following years. An event that contributed to the proliferation of the hotline centers was the suicide of movie actress Marilyn Monroe in 1962 – particularly the picture of her holding the telephone directly prior to her suicide. This tragic event focused major attention on the problem of suicide and raised public awareness of the crucial need for someone to talk to and the potential value of the telephone as a means of suicide prevention.

Emergency telephone services rapidly became a valuable source of suicide prevention and crisis intervention all over the world. Callers to these centers did not adhere to the original purpose, namely, suicidal crisis, but instead presented problems in a wide array of domains (Mishara et al., 2007), thus expanding the role of these centers in the field of community mental health to include the provision of emotional support and counseling.

The Unique Qualities of Emotional First Aid Provided by Telephone

Client Anonymity

People who seek psychological assistance are expected to open up to the therapist and disclose ultra-personal matters that may be associated with anxiety, guilt, fear, and other negative feelings. This requirement may be too threatening since it increases the feelings of inadequacy and helplessness. The help-seekers' ability to discuss personal feelings and experiences without exposing their identity may eliminate the barriers, there by affording a secure emotional environment in which they may feel free to share their innermost feelings.

Client Control

The client–therapist encounter is inherently inequitable since it is characterized by a discrepancy in power. The client is the one who requires assistance, who has fewer personal resources, who is at the mercy of the other party, and who is expected to disclose his/her weaknesses and shortcomings to an unfamiliar person. Since this situation may be embarrassing and even humiliating, it may discourage many individuals in distress from seeking psychological help.

Use of Trained Volunteers

The use of trained volunteers for purposes of crisis intervention and suicide prevention emerged in the 1960s as part of the nonprofessional revolution in the helping sciences whereby less-trained individuals were given roles in all areas of health, educational, social, and humanitarian fields. Nonprofessionals were being utilized in the growing field of crisis intervention more than in any other field (Heilig, Farberow, Litman & Shneidman, 1968).The rationale for using volunteers in therapeutic interventions was posited by mental health professionals who claimed that some of the problems people face can be handled better by trained volunteers because of the nature of the problem and the nature of the helper. For instance, Caplan (1964), who developed the theory and practice of crisis intervention, argued that individuals in acute crises who are struggling with a here-and-now drama do not require expertise in professional technique, but rather the assistance of someone who can provide immediate warmth, personal involvement, genuineness, and decisive direction. Such behaviors may be manifested easily and spontaneously by non-professionals who receive the proper training.

Non-professional volunteers have another advantage, namely, their ability to minimize the stigma associated with seeking psychological assistance. The latter is viewed by many individuals as a sign of weakness, causing them to eschew seeking help to reduce their suffering. The nonprofessional helper allays the help-seekers' fears in this regard, thereby enabling them to seek the assistance they require.

Eliminating Barriers of Distance and Mobility

Many individuals who require psychological assistance do not receive it due to limitations of mobility resulting from physical disabilities or geographical isolation. Even if they do not suffer from psychological disorders, their emotional well-being may be seriously jeopardized as a result of extended periods of low social interaction, as expressed by one man: "I have lived so much inside myself for the last three years that I believe that I have forgotten even how to approach and talk with other human beings" (Williams & Douds, 1973, p. 83). The telephone affords this person the opportunity to experience social interactions and maintain his/her psychological equilibrium.

Limitations of Emotional First Aid by Telephone

Overuse of the Service

By definition, emotional first aid aims to achieve a short-term effect such as obtaining temporary relief from an emotional burden, experiencing a sense of social affiliation, being given encouragement, or receiving information. In many cases, individuals who call the helpline suffer from more serious psychological problems such as major depression, severe anxiety, post-traumatic symptoms, eating disorders, and other ongoing disorders. In order to cope with these problems successfully, it is necessary to receive professional treatment whose objective is to effect long-term changes and develop inner resources. Since professional treatment is often more expensive – both psychologically and financially – than emotional first aid, many individuals in distress may compromise by obtaining temporary relief and avoiding the challenge of effecting meaningful, long-term changes. This process results in a phenomenon referred to as "chronic callers" that is manifested in the large proportion of callers who use the service very frequently – sometimes several times a day.

Chronic Callers

There are several limitations associated with the phenomenon of chronic callers. First, the overuse of emotional assistance by individuals who suffer from continuous loneliness and distress can be viewed as an inadequate way of coping because it leads to dependence on external sources rather than the development of inner resources that enhance well-being and social adaptation. Second, chronic callers occupy the helpline, thereby reducing its availability to users who may genuinely be in need of immediate assistance. Third, interactions with chronic callers may increase volunteer burnout since they are less challenging and less rewarding than interactions with first-time callers (Lester, Brockopp, & Blum, 1976; Watson, McDonald, & Pearce, 2006).

Lack of Nonverbal Cues

Eye contact, facial expressions, physical proximity, and other nonverbal communicative means of expression play an important role in face-to-face communication between client and therapist. They enable the therapist to arrive at an appropriate diagnosis and help both parties deliver rich and accurate messages. It is a common argument among individuals that the face-to-face encounter is necessary in order to experience authentic human contact, and clients should therefore avoid seeking help from technologically-mediated services. In order to cope with this limitation, helpline volunteers develop heightened sensitivity to receiving and interpreting vocal cues such as intensity and intonation, which partly compensate for the lack of nonverbal cues.

Evaluation of the Effectiveness of Telephone Helplines

A major issue in the practice and research of telephone counseling services is the evaluation of their effectiveness. Some of the difficulties in this research field are common to all therapeutic interventions, for example, defining criteria for successful outcomes and developing valid and reliable instruments for measuring these criteria. The evaluation of the effectiveness of volunteer-based telephone counseling is further characterized by two unique difficulties, namely, caller anonymity, which precludes systematic follow-up studies, and the ethical code of many helplines that prohibits the recording of the calls.

Four approaches to evaluating effectiveness are mentioned in the literature. The first derives directly from the original purpose of the helpline – suicide prevention – and focuses on studies that examine changes in suicide rates as a function of helpline availability in the community (Lester, 1997). The major limitation of this methodology is the multitude of factors besides telephonic assistance that can influence these rates.

The second approach to evaluating effectiveness was inspired by the humanistic psychology and client-centered approach introduced by Rogers (1980). This approach perceives the helper's empathy as a major determinant of psychological adaptation and personal growth. The utilization of this approach to evaluate the effectiveness of helpline calls was based on the premise that high-level interpersonal skills such as empathy and acceptance result in effective interactions with callers. Studies deriving from this approach measured volunteers' skills as manifested in recorded calls or simulations. For instance, Fowler and McGee (1973) measured three dimensions of the volunteers' responses: (1) empathy, defined as the ability to sense the feelings of the callers and reflect them back; (2) warmth, defined as genuine interest in the caller; and (3) authenticity, defined as the extent to which the volunteer constructively expresses his/her true feelings and thoughts.

The third approach is based on the rationale that certain organizational and professional characteristics of the helpline promote its effectiveness. Three such characteristics were defined by Motto, Brooks, Ross, and Allen (1974): (1) the utilization of criteria for selecting volunteers; (2) the use of ethical codes; and (3) the tailoring of the service to the nature of the community in which it operates. Other characteristics include 24/7 availability, systematic training of volunteers, and supervision by professionals. However, while these conditions are necessary for effective helpline functioning, they are not sufficient to ensure successful interactions with callers.

The fourth approach evaluated effectiveness on the basis of product variables such as client satisfaction and changes in the caller's state between the beginning and the end of the call (Fukkink & Hermanns, 2009; Reese, Collie & Brossart, 2002). The advantage of this approach resides in the fact that it furnishes direct evidence regarding the results of the interactions. Its limitation, however, lies in the bias of the sample, since only some of the callers agree to participate in the study.

CONCLUSION

Emotional first aid provided by trained volunteers via telephonic communication is a unique service within the field of mental health. The conceptual model underlying this type of service is based on two premises. First, emotional support for individuals in crisis can be provided effectively by nonprofessionals who receive the proper training owing to their ability to exhibit spontaneous warmth, personal involvement, and decisive direction. Second, telephonic communication creates conditions that can enhance the efficacy of psychological assistance, particularly the help-seeker's option to remain anonymous, his/her perceived control during the interaction, and the high degree of availability and accessibility of the assistance. These premises were fully supported, as is evidenced by the world-wide implementation of the telephone hotline, which became a valuable source of crisis intervention and suicide prevention. One conclusion that can be drawn from the popularity of hotlines is the significant role that technology has the potential to play in the development of psychological assistance.

Chapter 2

Characteristics of Psychological Assistance via the Internet

Abstract

The online environment has a dramatic impact on the nature of interpersonal communication, particularly by increasing the level of openness and self-disclosure, breaching the limitations of time and space, and offering a variety of communication patterns (e.g., synchronous, asynchronous, individual, group). These features facilitate revolutionary developments in traditional mental health assistance in the form of a technologically-mediated relationship between therapist and client. The advantages of rendering psychological assistance on the Internet constitute the focus of the present chapter. In addition, the historical background of this increasingly popular service is presented, and empirical evidence of its popularity is provided.

Introduction

The following message was sent by a 15-year-old adolescent to an online support group (forum) operated by the Israeli Association for Emotional First Aid (ERAN). Since the forum is publicly accessible, anyone can post a message, respond to a message, or simply read the dialogue that develops in the forum ("thread") following the original message.

"The only way to be released from the Jaws of Life"

I don't know how to cope with the problems I face, so the only thing I can do is release my pressure and write it all in one place. I don't expect anyone to pay any attention to this message, but I'm sending it because this is the only place where I can talk about everything anonymously.

I am a 15-year-old boy. I get along with my friends. I have quite a lot of friends and I also have a girlfriend. But I have still not been able to find my place in the world. I don't understand why. I have good friends, good grades. As a matter of fact, I have everything a boy my age could wish for. But still, something is missing. I don't know exactly what it is, but I know that I have been thinking about suicide recently. I don't understand it, but a few days ago I heard on the news that adolescent suicide is common in Israel. The minute I heard this I felt connected to the idea and this is what has been occupying my thoughts lately. A few days ago, I saw a truck while I was walking. For some reason, I felt a need to jump into the road and just let it run me over. Maybe the presence of other people prevented me from doing it, but since this happened I have been thinking of ways to do it. I know I wrote that I have friends and I guess they'll miss me if I do it, but for how long? We are still young, and I'm surely not that important to them at this stage of their lives. And what about my girlfriend? Will she miss me? I know she loves me very much and I love her too, but is it enough? They always say that love is not enough, so there's nothing real to keep me here. After all, the world will keep on going even without me, so why does it make a difference whether I live or die? In the end, everyone dies, so does it matter if I die a little earlier than when I'm supposed to?

I know that anyone who reads this message will think: 'What? Is he crazy? Why does he think about such a thing at this young age? His whole life is ahead of him.' I know that this is what it looks like, but believe me, it's not like that. I view life from a different perspective than most kids my age. I think that life is just a phase and death is another phase. I don't believe in life after death but I do believe that life has to come to an end sometime. So let's say that I don't feel comfortable now; why not be ahead of my time and move to the next phase? After all, my friends will eventually join me, so it doesn't really matter when I die.

I don't expect anyone to understand me, but I'm asking you to think about what I've written and try to understand me and my point of view. I'm sure that you will understand me, and maybe it will give a slightly different point of view about life and about the role we all have in this place we call 'Earth'."

In his post, the boy disclosed very personal aspects of his inner world. He chose the online group as an appropriate environment for sharing his thoughts about the meaning of life in general and his doubts regarding his own life – thoughts and doubts that extend to suicidal fantasies. The choice of the online group for the purpose of such profound self-disclosure seems surprising. It is reasonable to assume that an individual who decides to share his/her personal emotions and experiences will choose a familiar and intimate environment that offers the emotional safety necessary for this behavior. This boy, however, chose a group of anonymous individuals he had never met; he was totally oblivious to their attitudes toward the post in which he invested so many emotional and cognitive resources.

Why did he choose to send his message to an online support group? Why do millions of people who experience distress and seek understanding, encouragement, and advice, opt to seek assistance in an anonymous environment that is devoid of a face-to-face encounter and in which relationships are formed via written texts rather than by spontaneous speech? How can we explain the phenomenon whereby from the very inception of the Internet, surfers employed it as an environment for receiving emotional assistance, preferring it to the traditional agents of help in which communication is face-to-face? What underlies the attractiveness of the Internet to people who seek psychological assistance? The present chapter examines these questions and offers insights based on empirical studies as well as on knowledge that has been amassed in the last three decades regarding the practice of psychological assistance via the Internet.

Historical Background

The Internet is assumed to have revolutionized psychological assistance by creating conditions in which two parties who do not see each other can establish a relationship. In fact, technologically-mediated psychological assistance existed long before the Internet became a player in the arena of interpersonal communication, even though its use was limited and applied solely for specific therapeutic purposes. The first channel used for therapy was letter-writing. This counseling technique was employed by Freud, who wrote to the father of "Little Hans", advising him how to deal with his son (Freud, 1959).

The use of the telephone for rendering mental health assistance enabled a new model of therapeutic intervention to be developed, namely, emotional first aid provided by trained volunteers, originally developed for the purposes of crisis intervention and suicide prevention. The features of telephonic communication, particularly the option of anonymity and the high availability of assistance, contributed to its increasing success as a unique agent of help (see Chapter 1). The expansion of the telephone service to the online environment was natural since the two media share similar characteristics.

The use of the Internet for providing psychological assistance originates in the onset of the online environment; there is evidence of such usage as long ago as the 1970s. The first application used for counseling was probably a forum, which is an electronic bulletin board that can be used for posting messages and responding to them. This technological environment, which enables group interaction, was already used by self-aid groups when local networks of communication were operating. With the development of national networks, self-aid groups were open to all Internet surfers (Fink & Colon, 1999). The first forums presented experts' answers to questions posted by the users, an example being the well-known forum, “Ask Uncle Ezra”, which opened at Cornell University (the forum was named after Ezra Cornell, the University's founder) and provided responses to students' questions regarding mental health issues. Over the years, many online forums began to operate, adopting the model of face-to-face self-aid groups that has constituted a major means of social support for over a century. The participants in these groups were invited to share their experiences and emotions with others, as well as receive emotional support, information, encouragement, and practical advice (Stoney, 1998).

The use of the online environment by mental health professionals was probably initiated spontaneously by therapists who utilized the online environment to assist them in various ways such as employing email as an additional channel of communication with their clients and supervisors. Psychological assistance by professionals exclusively on the Internet began during the 1990sin the form of single-session consultations on specific issues. An example of this is the website of Ivan Goldberg, who began responding to questions online about the medical treatment of depression as early as 1993. Fee-based mental health services began to appear on the Internet in 1995. Initially, most of them offered to answer one question for a small fee. The earliest such service was offered by Leonard Holmes, who rendered psychological assistance by answering questions on a “pay if it helps” basis. Holmes reported that as soon as he set up a website advertising his practice, he began to receive emails from people seeking help. A later development was "e-therapy", in which the therapy strove to establish longer-term, ongoing helping relationships, all communication occurring only via the Internet.

A milestone in the development of online assistance was the formation of organizations seeking to integrate this type of assistance into the therapy establishment. The first was the International Society for Mental Health Online (ISMHO), a nonprofit organization formed in 1997 to promote the understanding, use, and development of online communication, information, and technology for the international mental health community. The ISMHO afforded e-therapists opportunities for receiving peer support, participating in professional discussions, and undergoing supervision. In the late 1990s, professional organizations of mental health therapists such as the American Psychological Association (APA) and the American Counseling Association (ACA) published ethical instructions for providing therapy via the Internet.

Emotional first aid provided by trained volunteers via the telephone was expanded to the online environment at the beginning of the 1990s. The pioneers of online assistance by trained volunteers were the Samaritans, who utilized email for the purpose of suicide prevention (Wilson & Lester, 2002).The expansion of telephone assistance into Internet assistance was natural and widely implemented, utilizing various technological applications and offering crisis intervention and emotional support (Barak, 2007; Fukkink & Hermanns, 2009; Gilat & Shahar, 2007).

The Advantages of the Internet for Psychological Assistance

The following texts were written by students who received counseling on the Internet and were requested to reflect on their online experiences as compared to their face-to-face experiences in a qualitative study on online counseling (Haberstroh, Duffey, Evans, Gee & Trepal, 2007).

> "It was little bit more comfortable, in a sense, talking to her. Because I know I never have to meet her. If I had something real big to talk to somebody about, that might be the way. Sometimes it's harder to face somebody when you have somebody looking at you. It makes it a little easier when you have that computer to look at and not somebody" (p. 275).
>
> "I kind of like the fact that typing in my response, it gives me a minute to think about what I'm going to say, and organize it. Whereas just back and forth, sometimes it's hard to come up with the words, and you stutter and you pause. Whereas in typing you just put down what you want to say" (p. 277).

> "It actually made it very comfortable for me. I really liked it. I got up that morning and took a shower and was still in my robe and I was able to sit down and have a counseling session. Whereas if I went to an office, I would be very concerned about my appearance, especially for that initial meeting. Making sure I was dressed appropriately, and I had my makeup done and my hair was done" (p. 277).

These quotations illustrate various advantages of interpersonal communication on the Internet and explain the latter's attractiveness to individuals in distress who need help but shy away from receiving face-to-face services. The literature suggests a number of characteristics that enhance people's willingness to seek assistance on the Internet.

Self-disclosure

The most salient characteristic of the interpersonal communication on the Internet is the elimination of the barriers that inhibit individuals from freely describing their experiences in face-to-face communication. The online environment is experienced as less threatening than face-to-face interactions, inviting the surfers to freely express their emotions, thoughts, and other aspects of their inner personal world. Several characteristics of the online environment combine to create a unique experience described by John Suler in the following words: "Everyday users on the Internet – as well as clinicians and researchers – have noted how people say and do things in the cyberspace that they wouldn't ordinarily say and do in the face-to-face world. They loosen up, feel less restrained, and express themselves more openly. So pervasive is the phenomenon that a term has surfaced for it: the online disinhibition effect" (2004, p. 321).

The disinhibition effect has two faces, one of which significantly enhances the processes of psychological assistance while the other can impair them. The first face is manifested in the willingness of individuals to disclose personal layers of their minds and share hidden feelings and secret desires that they dare not express in their direct face-to-face conversations with others. They exhibit compassion, kindness, and generosity, and expend a great deal of effort in order to help others, even if they are complete strangers. The online environment enables people to be in touch with their real selves, to experience intimacy with other human beings, and to freely express these intra- and interpersonal experiences. In terms of humanistic psychology, the online environment can be viewed as facilitating conditions that elicit the "real self" (Rogers, 1951). This kind of experience has a direct therapeutic impact in that it enables individuals to liberate themselves from the bondage of social desirability and develop their own selves.

The second face of the disinhibition effect is manifested in coarse language, unbridled criticism against others, verbal aggression, rage and hostility, and even threats. While this face is also rooted in the experience of disinhibition, it elicits the dark parts of the human mind, which are normally restrained in face-to-face interactions.

The high degree of willingness on the part of individuals who seek assistance on the Internet to be open and disclose their inner selves can be explained by the facts that they are neither seen nor heard by others and can maintain (almost) complete anonymity. They do not have to waste mental energy on their appearance and its possible effect on those with whom they are communicating. Moreover, external characteristics such as gender, race, age, apparel, and physical disfigurements, which highlight social differences between human beings, totally disappear. This engenders an atmosphere of equality and reduces the inconvenience and even threat experienced by those who consider seeking face-to-face assistance.

The option of remaining anonymous reduces the potential threat of being perceived as weak, dependent, and helpless by the environment. It also liberates the surfers from their commitment to their identity and enables them to build a new identity that is more consistent with their role as help-seekers.

The potential impact of anonymity on the willingness of individuals to disclose their personal experiences did not begin with the development of the online environment, and is reported in situations such as the phenomenon dubbed "strangers in the train". Rubin (1975) reports that complete strangers who meet in the train tend to share personal experiences (that they have never revealed to the people in their familiar environment) with their fellow passengers. Empirical evidence regarding the impact of the online environment on self-disclosure and the establishment of intimacy was presented in a study comparing two groups of participants who were requested to engage in a personal chat with a partner. In one group, the two partners were anonymous, and in the second, they knew each other. The results showed that the anonymous couples exhibited a higher degree of willingness to meet again than the couples who were acquainted (Bareket-Bojmel & Shahar, 2011).

The Use of Imagination

In every interpersonal interaction, we construct the image of the person with whom we interact and we engage in a dialogue with the image we have created of that person. The image construction process is based on the integration of external cues (the person's features) with personal meanings that we ascribe to these cues. In face-to-face communication, we are exposed to a wide variety of cues such as the physical appearance of the other person, nonverbal cues, and vocal cues (particularly intonation) that constitute the basis of the image and limit the need to complete it by means of the imagination. Since the online environment lacks visual and auditory cues, we inevitably use our imagination to complete the image of the ambiguous person. The construction of the image is not arbitrary; we project our own wishes, expectations, and needs onto the ambiguous figure at the other end of the online connection. This process of projection can explain the apparently surprising phenomenon whereby individuals develop very powerful emotional relationships (including falling in love) with people they have never seen. People who desperately crave love use their imagination to create the ideal figure that they want to love, and develop a relationship with that ideal figure. In the context of psychological assistance, projection can be very valuable because the help-seeker can shape his/her help-giver as kind, warm, and caring, thereby enhancing a helpful relationship.

Projection does not always involve positive emotions. People may project on their help-giver feelings of anxiety, anger, and hostility that they unconsciously retain in their relationship with others. This type of projection may be valuable in therapeutic processes, as Freud suggested in his concept of psychoanalysis. The client's hostility toward the therapist, which reflects the former's hostile attitude in his/her interpersonal relations, can serve as the core of the therapy. In the course of ongoing psychoanalysis, the therapist seeks to make the client aware of this irrational hostility in the hopes that he/she will no longer need it. Within the context of a single-session encounter with a trained volunteer, the projection of hostility or other negative emotions may jeopardize the helpfulness of the interaction. Managing these situations is one of the skills that volunteers are required to possess, and it is included in their training program.

Accessibility and Availability of Assistance

Communication on the Internet almost totally eliminates the limitations of space and time and therefore enormously increases the accessibility and availability of psychological assistance as compared to face-to-face and even telephonic communication. The elimination of geographical barriers may be particularly useful to people who require psychological assistance but are unable to receive it due to limitations of accessibility such as geographical distance, physical disabilities, or psychological barriers (e.g., social anxiety). The bridging of geographical barriers can be also helpful in face-to-face psychotherapies when one of the partners has to spend some time far away from the other. A unique advantage of bridging geographical barriers is evident in online support groups when the emotional experience of the participants occurs in real time despite the fact that they are physically located in different places – sometimes all over the world. This situation, which exemplifies Marshal McLuhan's vision of "the global village" (1964), may well create solidarity among the group participants and enhance the development of coherence and intimacy.

The Internet also eliminates barriers of time. Since the participants in the helping situations do not have to come to a common physical location, but rather communicate via their computers, communication can be immediate. This increases the availability of assistance – a particularly significant feature in situations of psychological crisis when the need for assistance arises immediately and any delay may have critical consequences. People who experience psychological crisis feel an urgent need to receive help and support in order to regain the emotional equilibrium that has been upset. If this need is not satisfied, they may develop more acute symptoms and their mental state may deteriorate. The high degree of availability of help is one of the major reasons for the success of telephonic hotlines as a source of crisis intervention and suicide prevention (Gould, Munfakh, Lubell, Klienman & Parker, 2002).

The degree of availability of assistance on the Internet is even higher than on the telephone thanks to the option of asynchronous communication. A person who feels distressed and needs social support can send a message to an asynchronous online support group at any time. Although an immediate response is not guaranteed, the knowledge that the message will be read and probably responded to by supporting others may serve as a source of relief.

Convenience

In face-to-face therapy, the client is expected not only to come to the therapist's clinic, but also to ensure that his/her appearance (appropriate apparel, physical neatness, and cleanliness) is consistent with the social norms for this kind of event. The online encounter enables the help-seeker to eschew the social commitment to "proper" conduct and appearance and behave entirely naturally – the way people behave at home. Moreover, the online connection reduces the psychological barriers resulting from various disadvantages such as physical handicaps, speech disorders, and so on that are common in face-to-face encounters. In addition, online encounters increase the client's control by affording a much more convenient opportunity to terminate the connection, should he/she wish to do so, than the face-to-face setting.

The Use of Written Texts

Although the Internet offers channels of communication such as video conferencing and Skype in which people can see and hear each other, in this book we focus on communication that is based solely on written texts – both synchronous (e.g., personal chat) and asynchronous (e.g., email and online forums). The therapeutic value of writing was recognized and demonstrated long before the Internet era. However, the dramatic increase in writing and writers that has occurred since the inception of online communication has raised professional awareness and increased the number of empirical studies regarding the potential of written texts for the purpose of giving and receiving psychological assistance.

An example of an "old-fashioned" use of writing for the purpose of increasing emotional well-being is the personal diary. A more recent example, which also included empirical support, can be found in the studies of James Pennebaker and colleagues (Pennebaker, 1997; Pennebaker, Mehl & Niederhoffer, 2003). Their studies were conducted according to an experimental paradigm, in which the members of the experimental group were instructed to write down their emotional reactions to everyday experiences, whereas the controls were instructed to write emotionally-neutral descriptions of their everyday routine. The results were dramatic, revealing a significantly higher increase among the experimental participants not only in subjective measures of well-being, but even in behavioral measures such as visits to the doctor. Following criticism directed at these studies, stating that they were experimental and could not be extrapolated to real-life situation, Lange and colleagues examined the effect of writing therapy on individuals who suffered from post-traumatic stress disorder. The structured therapeutic program that they developed, consisting of writing down emotional experiences and receiving feedback, yielded a significant improvement in the real patients' symptoms (Lange, Rietdijk, Hudcovicova, van de Ven, Schrieken & Emmelkamp, 2003).

One online arena in which writing plays a major role in describing emotional experiences is the personal blog, that is, the electronic version of the personal diary. The therapeutic value of writing in personal blogs was demonstrated in a study examining different types of blogs – emotional content vs. neutral content; receiving vs. not receiving feedback. The participants were adolescents suffering from social isolation and low self-esteem. The results revealed that the very act of writing, regardless of the content or the interactivity, improved the adolescents' sense of well-being. In addition, the most effective blog was the one in which the writers wrote emotional content and received feedback (Boniel-Nissim & Barak, 2011).

Emotional improvement is not the only positive outcome of writing in situations of psychological assistance. Writing has a major cognitive component, and some of the advantages are cognitive by nature. When expressing themselves in writing, people attempt to be more accurate, coherent, and organized than they are when they speak. This tendency results from the fact that writing is less spontaneous than speaking, and therefore the writer has time to prepare the message. In addition, unlike speaking, which is ephemeral, the product of writing remains documented, and the writer feels more responsible for its quality. The advantage of producing coherent messages is more salient in asynchronous channels of communication (email and online support groups) than in personal chats, which share similar features with speaking. A qualitative analysis of email interactions between distressed adolescents and trained volunteers (Rosenau & Gilat, 2011) revealed that both parties produced messages that were well-structured, comprehensible, and rich in linguistic resources.

Another advantage of written texts was demonstrated in the above-mentioned study, when the responses of the volunteers referred to all the topics presented in the sender's email. This could be achieved as a result of the full documentation of the messages. While writing their responses, the volunteers could read and reread the emails, thereby ensuring that they did not miss points raised by the help-seekers. Moreover, the responders quoted from the emails in order to reflect or to employ other strategies of emotional support. The documentation can be helpful not only to the responders but also to the help-seekers, who can reread the message, re-experience the emotional support, or hone their understanding of the cognitive messages or practical advice contained in the responses.

The Attractiveness of Online Assistance – Empirical Evidence

So far we have presented the theoretical rationale for the attractiveness of the online environment to individuals seeking psychological assistance. In this section, we present empirical evidence to support the theoretical arguments. Studies that examined the significance of the online assistance for both sides of the therapeutic encounter can be divided into two categories: (1) mainly quantitative studies that focused on the perceptions and attitudes of clients and therapists vis-à-vis the Internet as a therapeutic environment; and (2) mainly qualitative studies that focused on observing the personal experience of the participants involved in processes of online assistance.

In a survey examining the attitudes of Israeli adolescents toward seeking help on the Internet (Gilat, Ezer & Sagee, 2011), the subjects were presented with characteristics of the Internet that may affect an individual's willingness to seek psychological assistance. They were requested to consider each characteristic and decide how it would affect their own willingness to use the Internet for seeking assistance – in other words, whether its effect was enhancing, inhibiting, or neutral. The characteristics were as follows:

> "I can introduce myself by another name"
> "I communicate via written texts"
> "I can reread the interaction"
> "No one sees me or hears me"
> "I can leave a message at any time"
> "I sit alone in front of my computer"
> "I can provide assistance to others" (This characteristic refers to an online support group in which *all* participants can respond to distressful messages.)

The results revealed that all the characteristics were deemed enhancing, with only a minority of participants claiming that they were inhibiting. The characteristic that earned the highest percentage of enhancing influence was the ability to reread the interactions.

Another study examined the reasons underlying individuals' choice of the Internet as an environment for receiving psychological assistance. The option to remain anonymous received the highest score – 98% of the participants chose it as a motivating factor. This was followed by "convenience" – 71%. Interestingly, only a few responders chose "low cost" (Young, 2005).

A phenomenological study examined the experiences of adolescents who reported seeking help via the Internet as well as via face-to-face services and telephone helplines (King et al., 2006). A content analysis of their responses revealed three types of advantages of the Internet. The most salient was the emotional safety afforded by the online environment as compared to the face-to-face and telephonic services. The second advantage was the use of written texts, which provide a sense of protection from the negative feelings of the therapist. Finally, asynchronous communication gave them time to process the messages they had received and prepare their responses.

The experiences of adults who underwent psychotherapy conducted via the online environment were analyzed by Leibert, Archer, Munson, and York (2006). The major advantage was the psychological convenience of disclosing personal thoughts and emotions, particularly at the beginning of their relationship with the therapist.

How are the characteristics of the online environment viewed by the individuals on the other side of the therapeutic encounter? Like the clients, the helpers also perceive the characteristics of the Internet as enhancing the helpfulness of the therapy. Unlike the patients, however, the practical benefits received higher scores than the psychological advantages. Studying the attitudes of professionals toward online therapy, Powell (1998) found that the most frequently-mentioned advantage was the high degree of accessibility of the therapy for individuals who could not receive it due to geographical or physical barriers. The second most frequently-mentioned advantage was the option to remain anonymous, which affords the client emotional safety and reduces the tendency to behave defensively in the relationship with the therapist.

The above-mentioned findings were corroborated in a study conducted eight years later (Chester & Glass, 2006) in which online therapists noted the elimination of geographical barriers as the most frequent advantage. Additional advantages were the clients' low defensiveness and the full documentation of the interactions.

Another line of empirical evidence attesting to the attractiveness of the Internet for emotional assistance emerges from a comparison between the Internet and the telephone as mental aid media. This comparison can shed light on the unique value of the Internet owing to the fact that while some features are shared by the two media, others are more salient or occur exclusively on the Internet. Both the telephone and the Internet permit help-seekers to remain anonymous, increase the level of their control (as compared to a face-to-face environment), activate the imagination in the course of the interaction, and bridge geographical barriers. Internet communication is based on written texts, the degree of anonymity is higher (since people are not heard), and the variety of communicative environments (such as personal chat, online group, email) is much wider as compared to the telephone.

Studies comparing the two media as regards help-seeking were conducted by the Israeli Association for Emotional First Aid (ERAN), a volunteer-based mental health service that offers emotional first aid via the telephone and the Internet. A comparative analysis of the characteristics of calls to the two media revealed a dramatic difference between them –namely, the age of the help-seekers (Gilat, 2010). Whereas only 8% of the calls to the telephone helpline were made by young callers (under 25), this age group comprised 67% of the Internet help-seekers. A closer examination revealed that while children and adolescents (under 18) avoid seeking help via the telephone (only 2% of the calls were received from this group), a large proportion of them use the Internet (34% of the users belong to this age group). The attractiveness of the Internet as an environment for emotional assistance is particularly significant due to the low degree of willingness of many adolescents to seek help from formal agents. Studies show that over 50% of adolescents who suffer from acute distress avoid seeking professional help (Garland & Zigler, 1994; Offer, Howard, Schonert & Ostrov, 1991). There are indications that adolescents at risk exhibit a high degree of willingness to seek help from the Internet (Gould et al., 2002). The Internet can help reduce the gap between adolescents' need for mental aid and the actual use of face-to-face services.

The difference between the two media was not limited to age but was also evident in the nature of the problems presented by the clients. A study examining the proportion of suicidal cries for help on the two media found that 2% of the calls to the ERAN telephone helpline came from suicidal individuals, whereas 15% of all messages to the online support group were suicidal (Gilat & Shahar, 2007).

CONCLUSION

The online environment sparked a revolution in the field of psychological assistance by eliminating the barriers of time and distance and by facilitating anonymous encounters between help-seeker and help-giver by means of the transmission of texts. This revolutionary setting for psychological assistance is consistent with the principles and practice of volunteer-based emotional first aid, whose objective is to provide any individual who is experiencing distress in any psychological domain with immediate support. It is hardly surprising that volunteer-based emotional first-aid services evolved on the Internet as a natural extension of the traditional telephone hotlines. The online services have unique advantages that may help expand the populations who receive psychological assistance and reduce the gap between the need for emotional assistance and the availability of services to meet this need.

Chapter 3

WHO SEEKS HELP ONLINE? A STATISTICAL PROFILE

ABSTRACT

The purpose of the present chapter is to create a profile of the individuals who seek emotional first aid from trained volunteers on the Internet. Two components of the profile are presented: the characteristics of the individuals who choose to seek help in this unique environment, and the characteristics of the problem domains that these individuals present to the volunteers. In order to create the profile, we conducted a survey of 600 naturally-occurring online interactions retrieved from the database of the Israeli Association for Emotional First Aid (ERAN) – 200 interactions in each of the three channels that ERAN offers to the Israeli public: personal chat, email, and an online support group. The data were analyzed by means of a standard form that measured the following categories: gender and age of the help-seeker, type of assistance expected, problem domain, and suicidal crisis. The results revealed that two-thirds of the appeals for help came from females, and that the most prevalent age-group consisted of adolescents, even though young adults were also highly represented. As regards the content of the interaction, the most frequent problem domains were interpersonal relationships, self-esteem, loneliness, mental pain, and depression, while the most frequent type of expectation was that of receiving emotional support. The prevalence of suicidal ideations among the online help-seekers was very high – about 25 percent!

A comparison among the three channels – personal chat, email, and online support group – exhibited similar characteristics. The statistical profile of the online help-seekers foregrounds the value of emotional first aid on the Internet as a unique source of assistance within the repertoire of services available to individuals in need of psychological assistance.

INTRODUCTION

One of the characteristics of volunteer-based emotional first aid is the general nature of the assistance offered to the public. This signifies that anyone is invited to appeal for help regarding any problem domain. Many of the services that offer psychological assistance are selective by definition, that is, they target specific groups in the general population (such as youngsters, the elderly, or immigrants) or specific problem domains (such as violence, substance abuse, or eating disorders). The underlying rationale for offering a broad spectrum of assistance by means of emotional first-aid services posits that this is conducive to the creation of conditions that enhance the willingness of individuals to appeal for help. A 17-year- adolescent who experiences acute loneliness and needs someone to talk to does not have to consider whether her problem is consistent with the formal definition of one of the agents that offers assistance; she simply has to enter the chat, send an email, or post a message to an online support group.

In view of the general nature of the assistance offered to individuals who seek emotional first aid online, an empirical examination of the actual profile of the help-seekers and of the types of problems presented by them can be valuable from both the theoretical and the practical points of view. This study can shed light on the unique role played by emotional first aid via the Internet as an agent of psychological assistance. For instance, if we find that the population of help-seekers is characterized by a wide variety of socio-cultural characteristics, it will teach us that the service is viewed as suitable for a broad spectrum of the population, whereas if certain groups are underrepresented, it may indicate that this type of service is not viewed as attractive by certain segments of the population.

Most of the studies that examined the characteristics of calls to emotional first-aid services were conducted in the context of the telephone hotline (e.g., Gilat & Latzer, 2007; Gilat, Lobel & Gil, 1998; Lazar & Erera, 1998; Watson, McDonald & Pearce, 2006). The findings of these studies suggest some common characteristics:

(1) Females seek emotional first aid to a far greater extent than males; (2) The frequency of calls received from children and adolescents is very low

(much lower than their proportion in the population); (3) The problems presented by the caller represent a broad spectrum of domains, with loneliness and mental disorders as the most frequent categories. Other domains are identity-related problems, parent–child relationships, dating, sexuality, depression, and anxiety; (4) The prevalence of suicidal ideations and threats is not very high (considering the fact that suicide prevention was the original purpose of this service) – about five percent of all calls; (5) Hotline callers can be divided into two broad categories that differ with respect to most of the characteristics: chronic callers and first-time callers. The former expect mainly emotion-focused assistance such as listening and emotional support, whereas the latter expect instrumental assistance such as practical advice.

Empirical evidence pertaining to the characteristics of seeking emotional first aid from the Internet is scarce and limited to the domain of suicidal crisis. Studies have shown that many suicidal individuals seek help from online sources, particularly via email and online support groups (Barak, 2007; Lester, 2009), and they prefer the Internet to the telephone hotline (Gilat & Shahar, 2007). The attractiveness of the online environment to individuals in suicidal crisis is attributed to the disinhibition effect (see Chapter 2), which promotes self-disclosure and the sharing of ultra-personal thoughts and feelings with others.

This chapter presents the results of a study that expands the examination of online help-seeking. The main objective of this study is to create a profile of the seekers of emotional first aid on the Internet. An additional objective is to compare the characteristics of the help-seekers and the contents of the interactions among three online channels: personal chat, email, and online support group. While the three channels have several features in common, each one of them has a unique characteristic: the personal chat affords real-time conversation between two individuals – the help-seeker and the volunteer – and resembles face-to-face conversation the most closely; email is an asynchronous mode of communication that enables the writer to plan the messages and present them in a clear and organized manner; the online support group takes place in a group context, and the participants can benefit from the advantages of group processes. The comparison among the three channels will indicate whether the specific features of the communicative environment are associated with the nature of the individuals who seek assistance as well as the type of assistance they require.

METHOD

Nature of the Data

The sample consisted of 600 appeals for help that were received by ERAN's online service: 200 personal chats between the help-seekers and ERAN's volunteers, 200 email messages that were sent to ERAN's mailbox, and 200 messages that were posted on the online support group operated by ERAN. The data consist of naturally-occurring interactions that were automatically recorded on ERAN's website. Since this study focused solely on the help-seekers, we did not analyze the volunteers' responses. The sampling method consisted of the random choice of 200 texts from each channel out of all the texts that were recorded over a six-month period.

Instrument

A quantitative analysis of the texts was conducted by means of a coding form that was developed specifically for analyzing calls to hotlines. This instrument is based on a content analysis of interactions between hotline callers and trained volunteers, and was employed in studies examining the characteristics of calls to the Israeli hotline (Gilat & Latzer, 2007; Gilat, Lobel & Gil, 1998). In order to examine the applicability of the coding form to the analysis of interactions on the Internet, two of the authors analyzed 60 texts – 20 chats, 20 email messages, and 20 posts sent to the forum –in order to ascertain whether there were irrelevant or missing categories. This analysis demonstrated that the same form can be used for examining emotional first aid on the Internet.

The coding form consists of two parts: characteristics of the help-seeker and characteristics of the contents of the appeal for help.

Characteristics of the help-seekers consisted of five categories: (a) gender; (b) age; (c) family status; (d) occupation (student, soldier, employed, not employed); (e) history of mental treatment (reported, not reported).

Characteristics of the content of the appeal for help consisted of three categories: (a) type of expectation; (b) problem domain; (c) suicidal risk. Each of these categories is divided into sub-categories that are presented below.

Type of expectation from the assistance: Three types of expectation were defined, based on a content analysis of online interactions with ERAN's volunteers. The three types are not mutually exclusive, so that each one can be identified, independent of the others. Following are the definitions and examples of the three types.

Emotional support: The help-seeker wishes to share personal experiences in a supportive environment without any expectation of effecting a change in the situation. In many cases, this expectation is explicit (*"There's something nice about talking to someone you don't know. I don't have anyone to talk to in the entire world, except for you"*). In other cases, the help-seeker's expectation could be deduced from the content of the chat, the email, or the post to the online support group.

Instrumental assistance: The help-seeker expresses – explicitly or implicitly – a wish to change a stressful situation through the interaction with the volunteer. The nature of the change can be cognitive (e.g., adopting a less threatening and more optimistic view of the situation, gaining new insights into a perplexing situation), practical (e.g., receiving practical ideas for solving a problem), or both, as is illustrated in the following message posted to the online support group:

"I am a 16-year-old boy, living with my parents and brothers [...] I am having a bad time, there are a lot of things on my head that cause anger and anxiety [...] I am not satisfied with my life, I don't feel like doing anything at all [...] I want to change my life but I don't know how. Can you help me?"

Receiving information: The help-seeker asks for information – sometimes formal information such as mental health services (*"Where can I get professional therapy free of charge?"*), and sometimes professional information (*"I lost my sister two days ago and I can't cry. Is this normal?"*)

Domain of the problem presented by the help-seeker: Four general categories of problem domain were utilized in order to analyze the data: intra-personal problems, interpersonal problems, environmental problems, and mental problems. Each of these categories was subdivided into more specific sub-categories. The sub-categories included in the general category of "mental problems" indicate the nature of the problem directly, for instance "depression", "anxiety", "eating disorders", and so on. As regards the other three general categories, the sub-categories indicate a domain, such as parent–child relationships and the problems related to this domain, such as physical violence. The list of sub-categories is presented below:

Intra-personal problems: loneliness, self-esteem, identity, reaction to loss;

Interpersonal problems: spousal relationships, parent–child relationships, emotional distress, social relationships, sexual abuse, physical violence, sexuality;

Environmental problems: studies, work, unemployment, military service, economic situation;

Mental problems: anxiety, reaction to trauma, depression, eating disorders, schizophrenia.

Most of the sub-categories of "mental disorders" can be found in psychiatric classifications such as DSM. "Mental pain" is exceptional in that it is not recognized as a diagnostic category. It is a clinical concept suggested by Shneidman (1996), who viewed it as an acute mental state manifested by a mixture of negative feelings such as depression, anxiety, hopelessness, and loneliness. We added "mental pain" to the list of problems because in many cases, the help-seeker's problem could not be classified on the basis of the conventional categories. An illustration of mental pain can be found in the following message posted to ERAN's online support group by a young woman who expressed her mental pain in a poetic manner:

> "Why, God – why? Why aren't you willing to take me now?!
> I am tired of fighting my impulses, tired of the emotions, the pain that possesses me
> I am tired of feeling depressed, I am tired of being obsessed
> I am tired of the downs, the hardships
> Even though I sometimes feel good, I am simply tired of it all, I've had enough
> I don't need what's good, Evil has taken me over
> I do not desire joy for I am overwhelmed by woe"

The sub-categories of problem domains are not mutually exclusive, so each one can be identified, independent of the others.

Suicidal risk: Three categories of suicidal risk were utilized in order to measure this aspect:

Suicidal ideations: A wish to die is explicitly expressed or can be deduced from other terms such as "I want to disappear" or "I am sick of my life." Example: "It's enoughhhh! I want to die. Nothing works in my life. How long can you go on living in a world that does not exist? I was raped at the age of 11, my best friend was killed, my friends talk me into using drugs. What do I have to live for? My world is falling apart."

Suicidal threats: An explicit statement of an intention to commit suicide. Example: "I just took an overdose of sleeping pills. In forty minutes I will lose consciousness and then my systems will begin to collapse and I will die at last. That's it. After four years of suffering, I have decided to put an end to it. I love you all and thank you for the help you gave me during this difficult time. Goodbye, G."

Prior suicide attempt: An explicit report about a suicide attempt that occurred in the past.

The sub-categories of suicidal risk are not mutually exclusive, so that each one can be identified, independent of the others.

In order to measure the reliability of the coding, a pre-test was conducted by two research assistants who were presented with the definitions of every category and sub-category for the purpose of rating them. Each research assistant coded a sample of 150 texts (50 transcripts of personal chats, 50 email messages, and 50 messages that were retrieved from the online support group). The raters were requested to decide whether the sub-categories –type of expectations, problem domain, and suicidal risk –could be identified in the text. The percentage of agreement between the two raters was computed. In two of the sub-categories of "problem domain" – identity-related problems and spouse-related problems – the percentage of agreement was less than 85, resulting in the exclusion of these sub-categories from further analyses. In all the other sub-categories, the level of reliability was satisfactory.

RESULTS

All the variables in the present study, with the exception of the age of the help-seeker, were measured on a nominal scale. The age was recoded into four groups:

(1) children and adolescents under 18;
(2) young adults – 18 to 24;
(3) adults – 25 to 64; and
(4) the elderly –over 65.

Two types of analysis were conducted. First, a frequency distribution of each sub-category was utilized in order to obtain a statistical description of the characteristics of help-seeking. Second, a comparison among the three online environments – personal chat, email, online support group – was carried out using Chi square tests so as to ascertain whether there were significant differences among them.

FINDINGS

Characteristics of Help-seekers

Gender: Figure 1 presents the percentages of female and male help-seekers in each channel and in the entire sample.

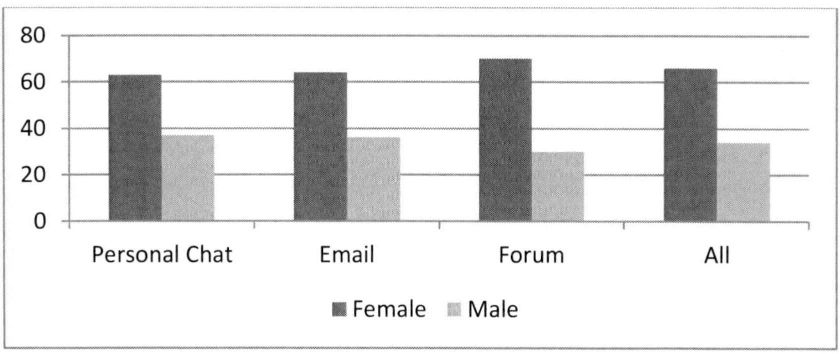

Figure 1. Frequencies of help-seekers according to gender and channel (%).

Figure 1 shows that there are almost twice as many female online help-seekers as there are males. The comparison among the three channels did not yield a significant difference ($\chi^2(2) = 2.65$, N. S.), indicating that the over-representation of females is characteristic of the online environment, regardless of specific channels.

Age: Figure 2 presents the distribution of help-seekers according to age group and channel of communication.

Figure 2 clearly shows that the vast majority of the individuals who seek online psychological assistance are young. Seventy-two percent of all help-seekers are under 25. About half of this group consists of children and adolescents, while the other half consists of young adults. Individuals who are older than 50 rarely choose the Internet as a channel for seeking assistance. Figure 2 also shows that the same pattern of age groups was found in all three channels, but the proportion of older adults (over 50) is higher in the email channel than in the personal chat and the online support group.

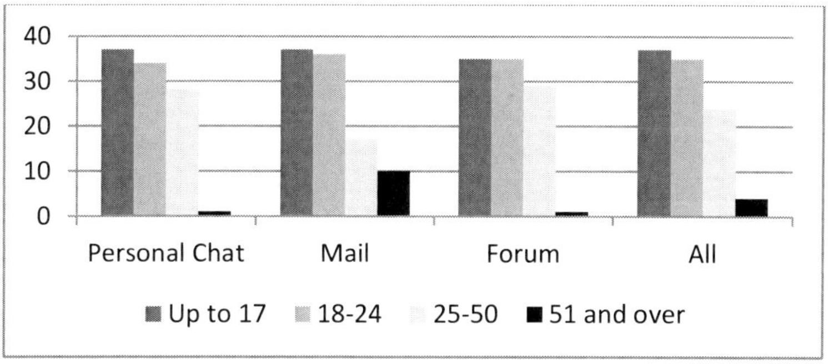

Figure 2. Frequencies of help-seekers according to age group and channel (%).

Type of occupation: Figure 3 presents the distribution of help-seekers according to type of occupation and channel of communication.

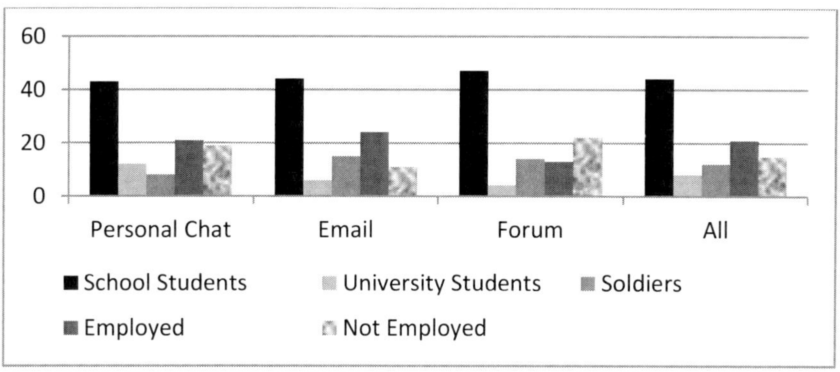

Figure 3. Frequencies of help-seekers according to type of occupation and channel (%).

Figure 3 shows that almost 45% of the online help-seekers are school students, about 10% university students, 20% employed, and 15% not employed (due to unemployment or disability). The relationship between type of occupation and channel of communication is significant ($\chi^2(8) = 31.54$, $p < .01$) as a result of a lower proportion of employed people and a higher proportion of people who are not employed in the forum as compared to the other two channels.

History of mental treatment: Figure 4 presents the distribution of help-seekers according to their history of receiving mental treatment (reported / not reported) and channel of communication.

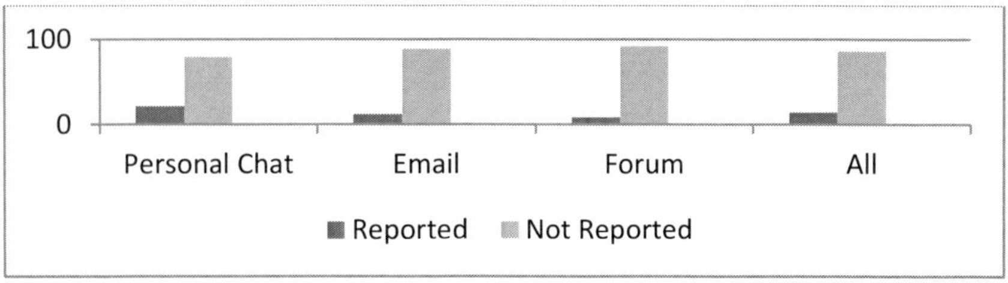

Figure 4. Frequencies of help-seekers according to history of mental treatment and channel (%).

Figure 4 shows that 14% of all online help-seekers reported having a history of professional mental treatment. A significant relationship between history of mental treatment and channel of communication was found (χ^2 (2) = 16.54, p < .01) as a result of a higher proportion of mental treatment among people who sought assistance via the synchronous mode of communication (personal chat) than via the asynchronous modes – email and online support group.

To sum up, the analysis produces the following portrait of individuals who seek emotional assistance online. Most of the help-seekers (more than two-thirds) are females. Since children, adolescents, and young adults constitute the majority of the help-seekers, most of the latter belong in a formal setting such as a school or the military. In addition, about 15% of those who seek help online also receive professional treatment. This portrait is characteristic of each one of the three channels of online environment – personal chat, email, and online support group.

Type of Expectation from the Assistance

Three types of expectations were defined: emotional support, instrumental assistance, and receiving information. Figure 5 presents the frequencies of the three types in each channel and in the entire sample.

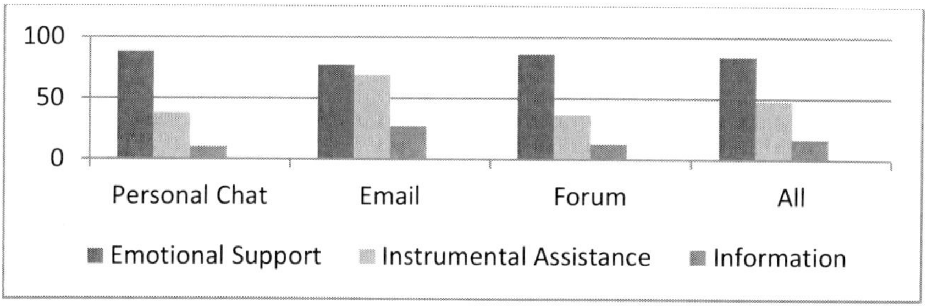

Figure 5. Frequencies of help-seekers according to type of expectation and channel (%).

Figure 5 reveals that the predominant expectation from the online assistance provided by the volunteers is emotional support, which is evident in more than 80% of the appeals for help. The wish to receive instrumental assistance such as practical advice was identified in almost half of the help-seekers, while the desire to receive information occurred much less frequently as compared to the two other types, and was identified in only 15% of the cases. The relationship between the expectation and the channel of communication is significant for each type of expectation. (Since the three types were coded independently, the test examining the relationship was conducted for each of them separately.) Receiving emotional support is more prevalent in the personal chat and the online support group than in the email ($\chi^2(2) = 9.52$, $p < 0.01$). Receiving instrumental assistance is significantly more prevalent in the email than in the other two channels ($\chi^2(2) = 53.99$, $p < 0.01$), as is receiving information ($\chi^2(2) = 22.41$, $p < 0.001$).

Problem Domains

The four general categories of problem domains were divided into more specific sub-categories, as described in the Method section. In order to learn about the profile of problem domains presented by online help-seekers, we computed the frequency of occurrence of each sub-category separately. As mentioned in the Method section, each domain was coded independently, with the result that the percentages do not total 100.

Table 1. Frequency of occurrence of each of the problem domains (%) (N=600)

Global category	Sub-category	Frequency (%) Present	Absent
Intra-personal problems	Loneliness	31	69
	Self-esteem	41	59
	Reaction to loss	7	93
Interpersonal problems	Parent-child relationship	32	68
	Emotional distress	54	46
	Social relationship	23	77
	Sexual abuse	7	93
	Physical violence	12	88
	Sexuality	4	96
Environmental pressures	Studies	11	89
	Work	11	89
	Unemployment	9	91
	Military	7	93
	Economic	5	95
Mental disorders	Mental pain	41	59
	Depression	28	72
	Anxiety	17	83
	Reaction to trauma	8	92
	Eating disorders	6	94
	Schizophrenia	5	95

The data presented in Table 1 indicate a broad spectrum of domains that were presented by the individuals who sought psychological assistance via the three online channels. Within this variety, there are certain domains that are much more prevalent than others. In the global category of intra-personal problems, self-esteem and loneliness appeared in more than 30% of all cases; within the global category of interpersonal personal problems, emotional distress (which includes painful relationship, loss of relationship, disappointment) appeared in more than half of the cases, and parent–child relationship was also fairly frequent. Within the global category of mental disorders, mental pain was extremely frequent (41%), and depression was also fairly frequent, occurring in almost 30% of the cases. The global category of environmental pressures occurred less frequently than the other categories.

In order to examine whether the three modes of communication differ with regard to the frequency of problem domain, we computed Chi square tests for each domain separately. No significant differences were found in most of the domains. Table 2 presents the four domains in which significant differences were found as well as the frequencies in each channel. The table presents only the positive frequencies (percentage of cases in which the domain was present). Since the measurement is dichotomous (present / absent), the negative frequencies are calculated as 100 minus the positive frequencies. For instance, if self-esteem occurred in 58% of all personal chats, it means that it did not occur in 42% of them.

Table 2. Comparison among the three channels regarding the frequencies of problem domains (%) (N=600)

Problem domain	Personal chat	Email	Forum	χ^2 (df=2)
Self-esteem	58	34	30	38.74**
Emotional distress in interpersonal relationship	63	59	40	27.66**
Social relationship	25	29	15	13.14**
Mental pain	25	47	51	32.16**

** $p < 0.01$

The results presented in Table 2 reveal that problems related to self-esteem were significantly more frequent in the personal chats than in the email and the online support group, emotional distress in interpersonal relationships and problems related to social relationships were less frequent among the online support group messages, and mental pain was more frequent in the two asynchronous channels than in the personal chat.

Suicidal Risk

As mentioned earlier, three measures were employed in order to study the prevalence of suicidal risk: suicide threats, suicidal ideations, and prior suicide attempts. The frequencies of these measures are presented in Table 3.

Table 3. Comparison among the three channels on the prevalence of suicidal risk, in percentage (N=600)

Measure of risk	Personal Chat	Email	Forum	Total
Suicide threats	26	21	29	25
Suicidal ideations	9	7	13	10
Suicide attempts	5	8	6	7

Table 3 shows that suicidal ideations were identified in 25% of the online appeals for help with no significant differences among the three channels. Suicide threats were identified in 10% of the total cases, and their prevalence was higher among the messages sent to the online support group than among the appeals for help via the chat and email. The difference approached significance ($\chi^2(4)= 3.85$, $p < 0.07$). Prior suicide attempts were identified in 7% of the total cases with no significant differences among the channels.

DISCUSSION

The aim of the present study was to create a profile of the individuals who seek emotional first aid on the Internet and to characterize both the domains of the problems they present and the types of assistance they expect to receive. In addition, the three channels of online assistance – personal chat, email, and online support group – were compared with regard to these dimensions.

The findings pertaining to gender differences revealed that women seek online assistance twice as much as men do, regardless of the channel of communication. This finding is consistent with many studies that examined the relationship between gender and help-seeking characteristics. Almost all the studies reported not only a greater willingness on the part of women to appeal for psychological help, but also the fact that they actually appealed for help much more than men. For instance, a meta-analysis conducted by Adis and Mahalik (2003) revealed that the more positive attitude of women toward seeking help traverses age-groups and cultures.

One of the more cited explanations in the literature for the gender differences is related to the social stereotypes of femininity and masculinity. This explanation claims that seeking help is more consistent with the social expectations from women than the social expectations from men (Garland & Zigler, 1994). In other words, men are less likely to seek emotional assistance than women because they perceive such behavior to be more threatening than women do. This claim should lead us to hypothesize that the gender differences with regard to seeking help diminish in the online environment since the anonymity of that environment eliminates the threatening connotation of seeking help, thereby encouraging men in distress to do so. Our findings, however, which reveal gender differences even in anonymous interpersonal communication, may be interpreted as showing that the social stereotypes of gender (particularly of masculinity) are so strong that they affect men's behavior even in a virtual social context. There may be other explanations for the gender differences in help-seeking on the Internet, but those explanations notwithstanding, our findings expand the generalization of the "gender divide" and demonstrate that it traverses not only age-groups and cultures, but also channels of communication.

As regards the age of the help-seekers on the Internet, the findings of the present study show that young individuals are over-represented. More than one-third of the appeals for help were received from children or adolescents. Another third came from young adults under the age of 25. These findings are not surprising in view of the ever-increasing role that the Internet plays in the life of young people. Since many of their social interactions take place on the Internet, the choice of this environment for seeking help is obvious. Their high degree of willingness to seek help from the Internet has valuable implications in light of the attitudes of this population toward seeking help from formal, face-to-face agents. Empirical evidence reveals that adolescents and young adults do not seek formal assistance even when they experience acute suffering. Studies on seeking psychological assistance assess the proportion of young people who eschew formal help to be over 60% (Offer, Howard, Schonert & Ostrov, 1991). This behavior is explained in terms of psychological barriers, particularly shame, as well as concern about the negative implications for their careers if their appeal for help is documented. Their willingness to seek assistance on the Internet is a result of the features of the online environment – such as the option to remain anonymous – which eliminate the barriers that prevent them from seeking help.

Interestingly enough, young people's willingness to seek assistance from the Internet is much greater than their willingness to use the telephone for this purpose. A survey on callers to the ERAN telephone help-line showed that 15% of the callers were younger than 25 (Gilat, 2010). The proportion of this age group among the online help-seekers, as revealed in the present study, is 72%. This finding implies that the attractiveness of the Internet for young people can be attributed not only to the option of remaining anonymous – an advantage that is offered by the telephone as well – but also to other features that render the Internet a unique and valuable source of emotional assistance.

Three types of expectations from the emotional first aid emerged: emotional support, practical advice, and information. The expectation of receiving emotional support is much more prevalent than the two other types, and it can be identified in the vast majority of the appeals for help. This finding is not surprising and is consistent with the main purpose of ERAN as a mental health service that offers emotional first aid. The comparison among the three channels with respect to the expectations of the help-seekers revealed the expectation of receiving instrumental assistance (practical advice or information) to be more prevalent on the email than on the two other channels. It is reasonable to assume that individuals in distress who require emotional support will opt for the personal chat, where their need can be satisfied [illegible]ediately, or the forum, where they can receive support from an entire g[illegible] mail's delayed response is more appropriate for giving advice or providing information because the volunteer has enough time to think of the appropriate advice or to obtain the information required by the help-seeker.

The problems presented by the help-seekers on the Internet represent a broad spectrum of domains, including problems of an intra-personal nature (e.g., loneliness, self-esteem), problems of an interpersonal nature (e.g., social relationships, parent–child conflicts), problems resulting from interactions with the environment (e.g., difficulties at work or at school), and problems that can be classified as psychological disorders (e.g., depression, anxiety, eating disorders). The wide variety of problem domains is consistent with former studies that examined the characteristics of appeals for emotional first aid by telephone (Gilat & Latzer, 2007; Watson, McDonald & Pearce, 2006) and is not surprising in light of the theoretical concept of ERAN. One of the principles that guide ERAN as an emotional first-aid service states that callers are invited to seek assistance for any problem that is bothering them, regardless of the domain. This principle aims to make the decision to seek assistance less threatening and more spontaneous, since the caller does not have to decide whether his/her problem is "suitable" for the mental health service. The main finding of the present study shows that this principle of generality is applied not only by callers to the telephone help-lines, but also by those who seek assistance online. This provides empirical evidence of the unique value of emotional first aid as a source of assistance for the entire population.

The various problem domains differed in their frequency of occurrence among the help-seekers on the Internet. Three domains occurred much more frequently than others. The most frequent domain was that of *interpersonal problems* such as social status, dating, and conflicts between friends, and was identified in more than half of the cases. Problems resulting from low *self-esteem* were identified in 40% of the cases. Problems related to *parent–child relationships* were identified in about one-third of the cases. The high prevalence of these domains can be explained by the nature of the online help-seekers: most of them are children, adolescents, and young adults. Individuals in these age groups experience numerous conflicts with their peers and their parents, and many of them are preoccupied with issues of identity and self-esteem. In many cases, the problems presented by the young help-seekers were not acute or critical, but rather represented everyday situations to which adolescents are exposed. The high frequency of these types of problems indicates that ERAN's online service is perceived as appropriate for the entire spectrum of problem severity and is not limited to severe psychological problems.

The above-mentioned finding illuminates the unique value of ERAN's online service as an agent of mental health. Many adolescents and young adults experience stressful situations that constitute an integral part of their particular stage of development. Although these situations are not severe enough to seek professional help (which is expensive both psychologically and financially), they impair emotional well-being and may lead to the deterioration of the young person's general functioning if no assistance is provided. The need for assistance may remain unfulfilled because the traditional sources of help are viewed as inappropriate: parents are sometimes the source of the difficulties and are therefore not the appropriate figures to resolve them; friends not only lack the maturity to be helpful, but are frequently occupied with their own problems; and teachers and school counselors are viewed as an unappealing source of emotional assistance (Gilat, Ezer & Sagee, 2010). Trained volunteers can eliminate this "service gap" (Raviv, Sills, Raviv & Wilenskey, 2000) between the need for emotional assistance and the willingness of the youngsters to receive it. Providing this assistance may be critical in maintaining psychological equilibrium and preventing deterioration in and permanent damage to their mental health.

In addition to the normative problems resulting from everyday stressful events, the online help-seekers also presented more severe problems that were classifiable as psychological disorders. The most prevalent categories of disorders were depression and anxiety, both of which were identified in about a quarter of all the cases. The type of assistance provided by ERAN in cases of psychological disorders differs from that provided to individuals who present normative problems. In the latter case, emotional support, encouragement, and empowerment may be sufficient to restore the psychological equilibrium of the help-seeker, with no further assistance required.

In cases of psychological disorders, professional therapy is necessary in order to cope with the problem effectively. There are various roles that trained volunteers can play in these cases. First, there are individuals who experience depression, anxiety, or other severe problems but avoid seeking help from professionals because they perceive it as too threatening. It is more convenient for them to seek emotional first aid. The interaction with the volunteer paves the way for professional therapy (Latzer & Gilat, 2000). Second, there are individuals who seek emotional first aid and receive professional therapy, but their need to share their feelings and experiences is not satisfied by the weekly session with the therapist, and they require another, more available, source of emotional support. Third, in some cases, the encounters with the therapist create emotional difficulties such as disappointment, hurt feelings, or anxiety for the clients, and they use emotional first aid as a means to process these difficulties.

The prevalence of suicidal risk was relatively high among the appeals for help via all three online channels. Suicidal ideations were expressed in about a quarter of all cases, and suicide threats were uttered in about one-tenth of all cases. The high incidence of suicidal crisis among the online help-seekers is not surprising and is consistent with reports in the literature about the attractiveness of the online environment to individuals who experience suicidal crisis (Gilat & Shahar, 2007; Lester, 2009). In the context of the present study, the prevalence of suicidal crisis in ERAN's online service can be explained by the combination of two independent sources. The first is the traditional linkage between volunteer-based emotional assistance and suicide prevention. The original purpose of this unique mental health service was suicide prevention (see Chapter 1), and it is still regarded as a major agent of suicide prevention owing to its characteristics, particularly anonymity and high degree of availability (Gould, Greenberg, Velting & Shaffer, 2003).The second source encompasses the characteristics of the online environment that reduce inhibitions and encourage the disclosure of very personal layers of the individual's mental world. Thus, individuals in suicidal crisis who feel an urge to share their mental pain feel more secure when they share their feelings in such an environment.

The attractiveness of volunteer-based online assistance for suicidal individuals is a valuable asset in the field of mental health, particularly for adolescents and young adults. On the one hand, this population suffers from psychological distress that can go so far as to engender suicidal ideations. Studies in the United States (Grunbaum, Kann & Kinchen, 2002) and in Israel (Tishby et al., 2001) show that about 20% of adolescents occasionally have suicidal thoughts. On the other hand, many of these adolescents avoid seeking assistance from traditional face-to-face professional sources due to psychological or practical barriers. The option to seek help in an online environment that eliminates these barriers eliminates the gap between the need for help and the willingness to seek it.

The availability of online suicide prevention services is particularly valuable in view of a dangerous phenomenon that increases the risk of suicide on the part of distressed individuals who surf the Internet. Since communication went online, the Internet has become a source not only of preventing suicide but also of encouraging it. There are websites that trigger suicidal behavior by glorifying and even directly encouraging suicide (Becker, Mayer, Nagenborg, El-Faddagh & Schmidt, 2004; Lester, 2009). This somewhat bizarre phenomenon has its roots in pre-Internet history, where literature and media reports about suicides exerted a powerful and devastating effect on those individuals who were struggling with seemingly unbearable mental pain (Etzersdorfer, Sonneck & Nagel-Kuess, 1992; Gould et al., 2003; Phillips, 1974).

The comparison among the three online channels with regard to the characteristics of the appeals for help revealed that the similarities exceed the differences. The gender proportion of 2:1 in favor of women was found in all three channels, and the distribution of age-groups was also similar, with young help-seekers (under the age of 25) comprising two-thirds of all cases.

As far as the problem domains were concerned, the high degree of variety was characteristic of all three channels. Only a few domains occurred at different frequencies. One of them was mental pain, which was more prevalent in the two asynchronous channels (forum and email) than in the synchronous channel (personal chat). Mental pain is viewed as an acute and unbearable experience. It may be so unique that individuals who experience it are not sure if others understand them. As a result, they require immediate feedback from their listener in order to be reassured that they were really understood. Such feedback can be provided via the synchronous personal chat but not via the asynchronous channels. Consequently, people who send distressful emails or post distressful messages to the forum exaggerate the intensity of their anguish in order to make sure that their message is understood. This explanation is supported by a study that examined emails sent to ERAN by adolescents. A qualitative analysis of the texts revealed that they employed a variety of linguistic resources in order to stress their pain, including verbal repetitions, overuse of words retrieved from the semantic field of negative emotions, and metaphors expressing pain.

CONCLUSION

This chapter focused on the characteristics of appeals for help addressed to an emotional first-aid service on the Internet. The findings afford a profile of the help-seekers, their expectations from the service, and the domains of the problems they presented. In general, female help-seekers far outnumber their male counterparts, most of the help-seekers are young, and the most frequent type of expectation is that of receiving emotional support. The problem domains are extremely diverse, with loneliness, depression, self-esteem, and social difficulties being the most widespread. The prevalence of suicidal risk was relatively high: suicidal ideations were expressed in about a quarter of all cases, and suicide threats were uttered in about one-tenth of all cases. In view of the fact that young people avoid seeking help from formal sources, the present finding implies that emotional first aid on the Internet can be a valuable asset within the repertoire of mental health agents.

Chapter 4

WHEN FACE-TO-FACE HELP FAILS: ONLINE ASSISTANCE VIA PERSONAL CHAT

ABSTRACT

The purpose of the present study is to explore the value of the personal chat as a source of emotional assistance for individuals who avoid seeking help from face-to-facc sources. Help-seekers suffering from Anorexia Nervosa (AN) and those experiencing trauma following sexual assault were chosen as participants in view of the difficulty involved in seeking face-to-face emotional help that is inherent in both disorders. We performed an in-depth, qualitative analysis on twelve transcripts of conversations between female help-seekers and trained volunteers that took place via the personal chat operated by ERAN. The analysis was based on the content of the conversations and on the discourse of the help-seekers. The latter disclosed experiences of unbearable emotional pain resulting from a negative self-perception, social disconnection, acute loneliness, and a strong belief that they were a burden to their families. In spite of their anguish, many of them avoided seeking either informal or professional assistance, and those who had appealed for help experienced disappointment. The personal chat, in which they communicated with trained volunteers by means of written texts from their own homes, enabled them to remain anonymous as well as to disclose their most intimate thoughts and emotions in a containing and supportive environment. The value of this experience is manifested in its ability to liberate them from an emotional prison and may also pave the way to professional therapy.

INTRODUCTION

The study reported in the current chapter presents an in-depth examination of the unique nature of online assistance by focusing on populations of help-seekers who experience acute anguish but shy away from appealing for help from traditional face-to-face agents. Such an observation enables the unique features of the volunteer-based assistance provided on the Internet to be identified.

The study examined two groups of help-seekers who sought assistance from ERAN: women suffering from anorexia nervosa (AN) and women experiencing trauma as a result of sexual assault. AN was chosen because of the barriers associated with seeking psychological assistance among individuals suffering from this disorder. There is empirical and clinical evidence showing that such individuals (most of them are females) avoid seeking both formal and informal assistance (Goldner, Birmingham & Smye, 1997). Moreover, even when they do consult a therapist, they exhibit a negative attitude toward the therapy, do not cooperate, and sometimes go as far as to sabotage the successful outcome of the encounter. This approach elicits a negative attitude toward the patients on the part of the therapists, which further reduces the possibility of a helpful intervention (Franko & Rolfe, 1996).

The fact that individuals suffering from AN avoid seeking professional help can be explained by an irrational decision-making process. The psychological threat associated with an encounter with a therapist is perceived as greater than the instrumental benefit from reducing the pain. Volunteer-based emotional first aid can be viewed as an attractive source of assistance owing to the anonymity, the sense of the client's control, and the interaction with volunteers rather than professionals. This attractiveness is supported by empirical evidence showing that adolescents and young women suffering from AN who called a telephone hotline reported that they had not appealed for professional assistance (Latzer & Gilat, 2000). Given all the advantages of the Internet as a communicative environment for people in distress (see Chapter 2), it is reasonable to assume that this willingness to seek help from the hotline will also be manifested on the Internet.

The second category of help-seekers examined in this chapter consists of women who were the victims of sexual assault. These women shared the characteristic of experiencing difficulty in seeking psychological assistance with women suffering from AN. Studies reveal that avoidance of turning to professional face-to-face agents for help is widespread among women who were victims of sexual abuse, and is estimated to be 70% (Campbell, Wasco, Ahrens, Sefl & Barnes, 2001; Ullman & Filipas, 2001). Several explanations for this maladaptive behavior have been offered: (1) The women blame themselves for the occurrence of the event and therefore feel unworthy of receiving formal assistance; (2) They neither trust the formal help-givers nor believe that their assistance can really be helpful; (3) The necessity to disclose the details of the intimate and traumatic event is extremely threatening because they are liable to relive the trauma; and (4) They are afraid that the help-givers will not fully believe their version of the traumatic occurrence (Patterson, Greeson & Campbell, 2009).

The present study was conducted using a qualitative methodology that was applied in order to analyze transcripts of naturally-occurring conversations via the personal chat of ERAN. The analysis was interdisciplinary, conducted by a team of researchers specializing in psychology and in discourse analysis. The psychological analysis aims (1) to identify the interpersonal processes that develop during the course of the chat between help-seeker and trained volunteer, and (2) to examine how the online environment affects these processes. The objective of the discourse analysis is to expand the insights regarding the psychological processes by identifying the linguistic resources employed by the partners in the encounter and interpreting them in the context of the present study.

METHOD

The Nature of the Data

The data comprised 12 transcripts of conversations between female help-seekers and trained volunteers that took place via the personal chat operated by ERAN. In six cases, the help-seekers presented themselves as suffering from anorexia, while in the remaining six cases, the help-seekers reported traumas resulting from sexual assault. Three criteria were applied for the purpose of selecting the transcripts: (1) The problem presented by the help-seeker (either AN or sexual abuse) was cardinal in the chat, that is, it constituted the focus of the chat and was not subordinate to another major type of problem; (2) The mean length of the transcripts was at least 2,000 words; and (3) Every chat was received from a different help-seeker (this criterion was necessary in light of the fact that many help-seekers are recurrent).

The personal chat is a synchronous (real-time) mode of online communication. The professional and ethical guidelines of this service are similar to the guidelines of all the other services provided by ERAN: the aim of the chat is emotional first aid and not professional therapy (see Chapter 1), the help-seekers have the right to remain anonymous while the volunteers are obliged to remain anonymous, and the conversation is discrete (i.e., no continuous relationship between the help-seeker and the same volunteer is permitted). Every chat is documented automatically and stored in a database. Since no visual or auditory cues are present, the transcript reflects the totality of the interactions that were studied. For ethical reasons, the pseudonyms that the help-seekers chose as well as their personal details have been altered so as to avoid any possibility of identification.

Data Analysis

The analysis of the transcripts was conducted by means of a qualitative methodology based on a data-driven approach. According to this approach, the analysis is not guided by predetermined categories, but rather is aimed at identifying themes that emerge directly from the data and can supply answers to the research questions. The analysis was performed by a team of three researchers – two of them mental health professionals experienced in online counseling, and the third an expert in discourse analysis. The analysis was conducted in two steps. The approach of the first step was holistic: each researcher read all the transcripts independently and identified general themes that emerged from most of the interactions. The list of themes suggested by each researcher was discussed by the team, and the resulting product was a list of themes that would serve as a basis for a more detailed analysis.

The second step was guided by an analytical approach: each theme identified in the first step underwent a further in-depth analysis. To this end, we reorganized the data according to the general theme; in other words, all the sections of the transcripts that featured a particular theme were grouped together. These new data units were analyzed thoroughly by means of a content analysis and a discourse analysis in order to obtain a detailed picture of the theme.

In the following section, we present the findings of the analysis. First we present the findings pertaining to the chats with the individuals suffering from AN, and then the findings relating to the help-seekers who had experienced sexual assault. The analysis includes quotations retrieved from the transcripts.

For ethical reasons, the quotations are partial and some of the help-seekers' details have been altered in order to prevent any possibility of identifying them.

FINDINGS

Eating Disorders

The help-seekers identified themselves as suffering from AN either directly –

> "I am anorectic"–

or indirectly:

> "... Everyone tells me that I'm too thin."

With the exception of one help-seeker, who was in her early twenties, all the help-seekers in this category were teenagers attending high school. They all presented a clear verbal description of their condition, suggesting that they were at different stages of the chronological development of the disorder. Three help-seekers began to develop the disorder shortly before making the decision to seek online help; they did not seek professional therapy from any other formal agent of psychological assistance. They did not seem to be fully aware of the significance of their condition. One of them, for instance, told the volunteer that her best friend had "forced her" to seek assistance from ERAN, threatening that otherwise she would report her friend's condition to her parents. The other three were more aware of the impact of their disease and they were undergoing professional treatment – either psychiatric or psychological. One of them said that although she had been cured, she was still afraid that the AN would return:

> "I simply can't get it out of my mind."

The major themes that emerge from the analysis are common to all six help-seekers: They were aware of the disorder, which they described as a "disease" and even "insanity"; they felt socially and emotionally isolated and positioned themselves as excluded from the social context in which they lived;

they devalued themselves and unleashed acute self-criticism that left no room for improvement or increased well-being in the future. In most chats, a turning-point became evident during the course of the interaction when the AN help-seeker began to heed the volunteers, who created an emotionally secure environment. She pondered the messages provided by the volunteer and espoused a somewhat more positive view of herself and a more optimistic perspective with regard to her future.

The major themes that emerged in the analysis will be presented below: the perception of anorexia, the self-perception of the anorectic individual, the help-seeker's positioning in relation to the figures surrounding her, how the help-seeker coped with the disorder in the past, and the value of the personal chat for the help-seeker.

Help-seekers' Perception of Their Anorexia

A major characteristic of the perception of AN is the awareness of its medical and mental implications. The anorectic help-seekers viewed themselves as suffering from a "mental disease" or "insanity":

> *"If Ana* [individuals who suffer from AN tend to personalize the disease, view it as a friend, and call it "Ana"] *can be called a mental illness, then I am mentally ill."*

Some described the disorder as a manifestation of insanity. This view is based on the response of the environment:

> "My family and friends shed tears and think that I've gone crazy",

and on their own view of normality:

> "It's not natural, and maybe because of that, I think of myself as insane."

Another indication of their awareness of the disorder is the need to receive help from external sources in order to extricate themselves from their situation.

A second characteristic of the perception of the disorder is an ambivalent attitude leading to an internal state of instability. This type of attitude was expressed directly –

> "I can't bear this instability any longer" –

and metaphorically –

> "...vacillation between the anorexia and the will to live".

The ambivalent attitude toward the disorder was further evident in the manner in which they coped with this burden. On the one hand, they adhered to the AN as a means of gaining control of their lives:

> "I know that I have Ana and I know that I am better than the other students in my class because they do not have control over their bodies."

On the other hand, they understood they were not healthy, they had a "mental disease", and they had to get rid of it:

> "I hate Ana when I give my food to someone else in school (I always have tasty food with me), but when I get back an empty plate and I know that I have succeeded, it feels good."

The ambivalent attitude toward the disorder was also evident in their perceptions of life and death. On the one hand, they expressed an explicit wish to die that is manifested in the rich use of words and terms related to the semantic field of loss and self-harm:

> "I wish I could die."
> "I want to cut myself";
> "I want to disappear";
> "I explode."
> "I know that if I commit suicide..."
> "I want to cut myself so badly."
> "I'm not succeeding in finishing myself off...I've tried everything."
> "I want to be small small small, lose weight until I die."

On the other hand, they revealed a desire for a normal and protected life:

> "I don't want to die, I want to live a normal and safe life."
> "I simply want to be normal."

The craving for a normal life was also implicitly expressed by means of questions such as *"When will this nightmare come to an end?"*

The internal conflict was also evident in the desire to be thin and the need to eat:

> "I'm sick of the efforts to maintain my weight and to lose and gain weight constantly."

Their discourse revealed that this intra-personal ambivalence also extended to the interpersonal context. One manifestation of this duality was the struggle between the need to conceal the disease from their surroundings, particularly from their parents, and the need to disclose their condition in order to obtain relief:

> "I hide my feelings but my problems become greater."

Another manifestation of the duality focused on seeking assistance:

> "On the one hand, I need help, but on the other hand, I'm very introvert and don't share my feelings with anyone, and I'm also too shy to tell them that I need help."

A third characteristic consisted of perceiving the disease as death and exhibiting an ambivalent attitude toward this death. On the one hand, they saw death waiting for them at the end of the road they were following and stated that they did not want to die, asking:

> "When will this nightmare come to an end?"

On the other hand, some of them viewed death as an escape from the unbearable agony they were experiencing at that moment:

> "It's better to die forever than go on suffering for an entire year."
> "I wish I'd turn into a stone."

This attitude is extremely dangerous when death is regarded as the only effective solution to their agony:

> "The only thing that would help me right now is a sleep from which I will not wake up."

The linguistic analysis shows this attitude to be manifested in words and expressions retrieved from the semantic field of death: "to die," "to disappear," "to explode," "a sleep of death," "suicide."

Self-perception

The chats permitted the creation of a self-portrait of the anorectic help-seekers that shed light on their identity as reflected by the environment in which they lived. According to Bakhtin (see Wortham, 2004), the identity developed by the individual emerges from social categories. The process of shaping the self-perception is rooted in social resources and therefore the self-perception is a reflection of the way in which the social environment perceives the individual. In all the transcripts that were analyzed in this study, there was a clear expression of the self-perception, which consisted of two components: physical and psychological.

Physical self-perception: The help-seekers understood that although their environment viewed them as thin, they were convinced that they were obese:

> "...They say I'm thin, but I don't feel that way, and it's frustrating."

They yearned to be thin so that they could like their bodies –

> "I want to get thin until I'm satisfied with my body" –

but in the meantime they did not like the way they looked in the least:

> "I am a cow, a cow."

Their appearance was of utmost importance to them:

> "More than anything else, I am interested in how I look when I look in the mirror."

They were caught between two conflicting drives – losing weight on the one hand and coping with the disorder on the other.

Personal self-perception: The most salient characteristic of the self-portrait that emerged from the chats was severe self-criticism and self-hatred:

> "I'm anorectic and I hate myself because of it."

They explicitly described themselves as worthless:

> "I am shit, I am boring, I am nothing, just nothing."

This self-perception was also expressed as a minimization of their selves:

> "I am a statistical cipher."
> "I want to be small small small, lose weight until I die."

The manner in which they were viewed by their surroundings, as reflected in their descriptions, was also extremely negative. They ascribed this point of view to their parents –

> "... Then my parents will understand that their daughter is dumb, that her life is superficial and focuses on diets" –

and to the broader environment:

> "I am viewed as disgusting and that is my problem. I am used to it, they always blame me, they always criticize me and show me that I am the most loathsome thing that has ever been created in the world."

In some cases, they wrote about other people in general, but they were probably referring to themselves:

> "Everyone is weak when they are alone, that's why people want to fit in and avoid showing their true selves. They are afraid of the criticism, they are afraid that society will ostracize them and they will remain all alone."

Positioning

The analysis of the chats clearly reveals the positioning of the anorectic help-seekers, that is, the manner in which they presented themselves in relation to other agents in their lives –their life-space, society, and their parents. Some of them positioned themselves in relation to their friends and their therapists. They all positioned themselves in relation to the volunteer, and this positioning changed as the chats proceeded.

Positioning in relation to life-space and society: The anorectic help-seekers described their life as *"garbage" or "the pits"*:

> "My life is in the garbage [...] I am tired of this life, everything is disgusting in this life."
>
> "I feel like trash, a big piece of trash."
>
> "Nothing is left, not a ray of light."

This view indicates a positioning of alienation, of shying away from life.

Their positioning in relation to society was also characterized by alienation and their self-imposed status as outsiders. A major component of their positioning stemmed from the conviction that no one understood them:

> "No one can understand how it feels to be me and no one is interested enough or tries to see what I'm carrying in my heart."
>
> "... nobody around me understands what's happening to me and why I behave the way I do."

They also expressed the discrepancy between their appearance on the one hand and their inner feeling on the other:

> "People see me friendly and smiling and they have no idea how I feel inside."

They perceived other people's attitudes toward them as ranging from indifferent to hostile. Another feature of their positioning in relation to their social environment was their perception of being a burden.

> "No one cares about me [...] I'm gradually understanding it [...] Everyone hates me[...] there is no one I can trust."
>
> "I feel that everyone around me would like to get rid of me if they only could." "No one would miss me and right now I am a burden to too many people."

Due to the alienating attitude of society toward them, most of them preferred to be alone –

"I am alone and I like it this way. I don't need any favors from anyone in this world"–

and listed the benefits of their solitary state:

"No one can upset me, there is no one to judge me, I don't need to hide [anything] or lie to anyone, there is no one to cry for me and no one to laugh, pretending to be happy just to make me feel happy."

Positioning in relation to their parents: In light of their alienation, loneliness, and social disconnection, they might be expected to view their parents as a source of support and encouragement. However, their positioning toward their parents, as reflected in the analysis of the chats, was in fact quite different: they endeavored to conceal their condition from their parents. They justified this approach by the need to protect their parents from having to face the burden:

"They are having a hard time anyway and I'll make it more difficult for them [...] I'll cause troubles in my family and I don't want this."

"No one knows how lousy I feel because they're suffering on my account. I feel bad that I'm causing this mess because I love them, I feel like I'm a catastrophe in the middle of their home, I'm ruining the atmosphere."

One of them even left home so that her parents did not have to see her and suffer because of her condition. In one case, although their parents knew about the disease and supported their daughter she considered her presence a burden:

"They give me support, but they are tired of it; how long can they suffer me?"

Positioning in relation to the therapist: Only two anorectic help-seekers mentioned their therapists in the chat, and their attitude toward them was ambivalent:

"I like my psychologist, he helps me during the sessions, but he can't be by my side all the time."

Subsequently she wrote:

"The therapy does not help me at all."

Positioning in relation to the volunteer: In all chats, a similar pattern of positioning in relation to the volunteer was identified. This pattern was characterized by a change in the attitude exhibited toward the volunteer as the interaction proceeded. It began with an expression of devaluation and apology on the part of the help-seeker, continued with a request for support and intimacy, and concluded with an expression of gratitude.

In most cases, the chat began with expressions of apology:

> "I'm sorry to bother you."
> "Are you there? I don't want to disturb you."

They knew that the volunteer was expected to give support, and yet they devalued themselves:

> "You don't really mean it. You said it because you don't want to hurt me and cause me more pain."

As the chat evolved, they began to change their attitude and attempt to establish a relationship by asking the volunteer to furnish personal details such as name, age, and gender. The desire to render the virtual relationship more concrete and to establish an intimate connection between help-seeker and volunteer was manifested in the request for a hug:

> "It's so difficult for me!!! Can you send me a hug? A protective hug, so that nothing will hurt me."

The intimacy was also manifested in the anorectic help-seeker's promise that she would not harm herself:

"Don't worry, I am alive, really, I am alive." (The aim of this statement was to reassure the volunteer following the explicit suicidal ideations that had been uttered during the course of the chat.)

The analysis of all the chats revealed a turning-point that altered the course of the process and induced the help-seeker to pay attention to the volunteer. This turning-point was characterized by a challenging comment directed at the volunteer, or some kind of wish that could be interpreted as a cry for help. The following quotation illustrates a challenging comment of that type:

Volunteer: I am discovering a wonderful girl, clever, mature...
Iris: I appreciate it very much, thank you.
Volunteer: With so many insights...
Iris: So I want to hear another insight from you.

Another help-seeker challenged the volunteer with the statement:

"Let's see if you can help me,"

while a third asked plaintively:

"What's wrong with me? Am I abnormal? What's the matter with me?"

Following these challenging comments, the help-seekers expressed their specific requests for assistance:

"What the hell am I supposed to tell my parents?"

"Do I need something specific against eating disorders or something more general?"

"Where do I find a physician who doesn't know my mother and won't tell her if something is wrong?"

"Is there any other possibility besides hospitalization?"

Most of the chats concluded with expressions of gratitude to the volunteer for being understanding and supportive:

"Thank you, really thank you."

"Good night, you really helped me."

"Thank you for staying with me for an additional half-hour even though you're probably dying to go to sleep."

"Thank you for putting up with me."

In some cases, the help-seekers mentioned a specific type of assistance that they received:

"You helped me arrive at several decisions and I'm even smiling, so thank you."

Another anorectic help-seeker sent an email, about a month after the chat, reflecting upon her experience during the chat and its impact:

> "He [the volunteer] made me feel at ease and made me feel as if someone really cares about me."

Following the chat, she decided to come to grips with the disease:

> "For several days, I repeatedly thought about the things he had told me that evening [...] a month from then, I am happy to tell you that I am succeeding. I must say that it's not perfect, but I eat, I don't vomit anymore, and my digestive system is becoming accustomed to the new situation."

Coping

The analysis of the transcripts reveals several strategies employed by the anorectic help-seekers in order to cope with the stressful experience resulting from the disease. These strategies can be divided into two categories: (1) adaptive strategies that might reduce their suffering and enhance their emotional welfare, and (2) maladaptive strategies that might not only fail to lead to positive consequences, but occasionally even increase the level of distress.

Adaptive coping: Two adaptive strategies were mentioned by the help-seekers, namely, applying for external assistance and mobilizing internal resources. Most of them told the volunteers that they were seeking help from a mental health professional, admitting that they were incapable of helping themselves without an external source:

> "I saw a psychiatrist last week because I felt that I couldn't cope all by myself." "I realized that I will never succeed in doing everything by myself and that I draw a great deal of strength from significant relationships in my life, even though it is hard to establish them. It's impossible to be alone. It doesn't work, it's too much."

Another help-seeker recounted that she had hospitalized herself and was receiving professional help:

> "I realized that my condition was very severe and went to a hospital. I was discharged about three weeks ago and I feel bad, very bad. I see a psychologist twice a week, and tomorrow I begin treatment with a dietician."

The mobilization of internal resources was rare and was mentioned by only one of them:

> "I tell myself that I mustn't break just because it is a difficult time. If it is too difficult, you take a deep breath and get through it like an adult."

Maladaptive coping: Several strategies that may increase the risk were mentioned, all of which had one feature in common, namely, avoiding the problem. Some of the help-seekers concealed the disease from the people close to them, particularly their parents:

> "There are people who love me, but I am very introverted and I don't talk to others about my problems [...] I don't believe they can help me and I'm also ashamed to tell them that I need help."

Others resort to drastic measures such as self-harm or suicide attempts:

> "I have been taking pills for more than a month, but nothing finishes me off... I've tried everything, I've cut myself, nothing helps."

Sexual Assault

Introduction

The chats analyzed in this part all involved female help-seekers who recounted an objective event in which they were sexually assaulted by a man. The timing of the event in relation to the appeal for help ranged from one day to seven years prior to the chat. All the help-seekers can be characterized as normative adolescents or women who had not suffered from mental disorders preceding the sexual attack; the unexpected traumatic event disrupted the balance of their routine and changed their lives dramatically.

Before contacting ERAN, almost all the help-seekers had sought professional assistance. However, since they felt that the encounter with the professional help-givers neither restored their peace of mind nor helped them resume their normal, routine lives, they decided to try the emotional first aid offered on the Internet. The unique features of the online environment in which their chats occurred, particularly the anonymity and the use of the medium of writing, enhanced their openness and self-disclosure. They shared with the volunteers the deepest layers of their experiences – something they had probably not done during the encounters with the professional help-givers in the face-to-face environment. This process enabled us, as researchers, to gain insights into their complicated and anguished minds, examine the inadequate coping strategies they had employed, and shed light on the unique value of the online assistance to their emotional welfare. The analysis revealed four aspects, which are presented in this section: (1) a view of the traumatic event; (2) the self-perception of the assaulted help-seekers; (3) their positioning vis-à-vis the environment; and (4) the coping strategies they employed.

Viewing the Traumatic Event

Three motives that are associated with the sexual assault emerged from the analysis of the chats:

The enormous significance of the event in the victim's life: All the help-seekers described the sexual assault as a major event that consumed much of their mental energy. In some cases, it was described as a turning-point in their lives.

> "I have something huge in my life that I never managed to resolve."
> "I was a different person, I changed so drastically, my thinking is different, I hesitate, I've never behaved that way."

The effect of the event on their level of functioning: The help-seekers described severe symptoms that were manifested in a variety of domains:

(1) physical symptoms – *"I feel that my chest is burning as if something is really painful,"*

(2) emotional symptoms – *"two weeks after it occurred, I was afraid to leave my home, even to throw away the garbage,"*

(3) cognitive symptoms – *"I simply cannot stop thinking about it. It comes out every second, it doesn't leave my mind,"*

(4) behavioral symptoms – *"... My school average decreased from 98 to 80. I stopped going to school because I couldn't concentrate, couldn't listen."*

One of them wrote the word "nightmare" three times in succession in order to abstract the impact of the traumatic event.

Avoiding the use of explicit words to denote the sexual attack: This linguistic characteristic, which is imbued with a psychological meaning, was identifiable in all the chats with sexually-abused help-seekers. One of them wrote "rape" in English (even though the chat was conducted in Hebrew) and added:

> "I prefer not to see this word in Hebrew."

Another help-seeker frequently used the word "that" instead of "rape". In another case, the event took place one day before she appealed for help and she wrote:

> "I am here because I was almost raped yesterday."

Another help-seeker wrote "rape" and explained that she preferred to put the word in brackets:

> "It seems to me more difficult to write this word without brackets."

Avoidance of the use of the word "rape" in an explicit way, without limitations and reservations, can be interpreted as an attempt on the part of the help-seekers to defend themselves against the emotional threat of the traumatic event, thereby distancing the experience from their awareness.

Self-perception

Several characteristics of the help-seekers' self-perceptions emerged from the analysis of the chats.

Hesitation, confusion, lack of confidence: One help-seeker related an event that had occurred seven years earlier. She identified herself in relation to this event by labeling herself "Searching for Myself". This label indicates that she viewed herself as indecisive, unsure of which measures to take with regard to the event. This self- perception of confusion and hesitation was also manifested in the frequent use of words and expressions retrieved from the semantic field of hesitation and doubt:

> "...I called after years of hesitation and fear of my own reaction [...] but I don't know how, I don't know how to talk, what to say. I don't know where to steer my head. I don't know if I should open things up."

Self-blame: The objective circumstances described by the help-seekers clearly indicate that they were the victims of sexual assaults – and yet all of them blamed themselves, at least to a certain extent. In some cases, the self-blame was specific, focused on the event itself:

> "I shouldn't have gone there."

In other cases, the self-blame was generalized to the victim's entire personality and viewed as a punishment for being a bad person:

> "I feel guilty and defective, I can prove that I am guilty."

The guilt was also reflected in the way in which she believed she was perceived by her surroundings:

> "I'm afraid that they [her family] will say that I was to blame because I went there and I did not object."

The feeling of guilt could be so strong that it led to self-criticism, the inability to accept herself, and the conviction that nobody could accept her the way she was:

> "Part of the fact that I can't tell others about it is simply because I can't accept myself...so how can I expect others to accept me?"

Need for help: Although most of the help-seekers had received assistance from a professional, they expressed a very strong and an immediate need to be helped. This need was explained by a mixture of pressure to "let it out", helplessness, confusion, doubt, and the inability to decide what to do, which almost drove them to distraction.

> "What am I supposed to do with this feeling now? I don't know what to do with it now."
>
> "I just want a way to cope with those thoughts, I want to talk about it, please help me."
>
> "Once I asked for help and now I'm begging for help."

Positioning

In light of the fact that parents are the most meaningful figures for their children, it is interesting to see how the sexually-abused help-seekers positioned themselves in relation to their parents. The analysis showed the major characteristic of this positioning to be the tendency to conceal the traumatic event from their parents. The help-seekers avoided disclosing the dreadful experience to them and went to great lengths to prevent them from finding out about it:

> "I don't want to tell my parents anything."
>
> "My parents are the last address, believe me."
>
> "I'm afraid that my parents will hear about it and I don't want them to be involved in it, not at all."

The decision to conceal the event from their parents stems from the latter's anticipated – or real – reaction upon hearing about the sexual attack from others, or, in rare cases, from the daughter herself.

In some cases, the parents exhibited negative responses such as anger, disappointment, and even blame:

> "... They are very angry with me because I went there [...] I am afraid that they're saying that it was my fault because I didn't leave the place immediately."
>
> "When they heard about it, the entire household was distraught and my parents didn't stop crying."

Even when the parents lent support to their distressed daughter, the assistance was instrumental and not emotional:

> "She [her mother] went with me to the police, but she doesn't understand that I'm still in a state of trauma."

The need to conceal the event is also evident in their relationships with other close figures such as a boyfriend:

> "I feel very safe with him, but if I tell him what happened, it will cause trouble."

Another aspect of their relationship with their environment that emerged from the analysis was the help-seekers' dichotomous approach. They differentiated between good, understanding, supportive, and helpful people on the one hand, and bad, dangerous people on the other. The "enemy" group comprised the psychologist at the emergency center, who reported to the parents, and the sister who accused the help-seeker of causing trouble for their parents. The "helpful" group was small, comprising the teacher who heard about the sexual attack and canceled a lesson so that she could talk to the help-seeker privately. The volunteers could also be included in the group of helpful people, as is evident from the grateful responses at the end of the chat.

Coping

The analysis yielded several coping strategies employed by the sexual assault victims before they sought online assistance. These strategies, however, were not altogether helpful in resolving the traumatic experience and enabling the victims to return to their normal, everyday routine.

Avoidance: The tendency to avoid taking direct measures in order to cope with the trauma was described as a deliberate decision to bury the traumatic experience / at the back of their minds:

> "I didn't reveal anything and I have remained closed up in myself."
> "I buried everything and didn't cope, so there was nothing for me to tell."
> "I didn't let it sit in my head, I simply repressed it."

Over the course of time, this wall of repression began to crumble, and the victims experienced internal pressure to share the traumatic experience and seek assistance. However, in most cases, the appeal for help did not produce the desired improvement; on the contrary – it sometimes actually increased the distress.

Procrastination: Procrastination is a strategy in which a person does not take the action that is needed in order to change a stress ogenic event, but rather postpones the action to a later time. This strategy is usually employed in situations in which the person feels helpless and vulnerable, with the result that operating proactively may raise the level of anxiety and decrease the self-efficacy required for successful coping. The procrastination strategy employed by the help-seekers was illustrated in the chats, particularly in connection with going to the police and filing a complaint:

> "I made myself a promise that I would file a complaint only when I felt confidence in myself. My self-confidence is very low right now. I can't stand the thought of standing in front of him [the offender], it will not be helpful to me now."

Appeal for assistance: Seeking emotional assistance, which is one of the most prevalent coping strategies, is employed by individuals who experience emotional distress. There are two types of agents who usually render assistance to help-seekers: informal agents, particularly parents and friends; and formal agents, particularly mental health professionals. Both types of assistance were mentioned by the sexually-abused help-seekers.

As regards the informal sources, it was surprising to find that parents were not mentioned as a source of support by the help-seekers. On the contrary – some of them perceived their parents as a source of tension, as described above (see "positioning"). The informal figures that provided emotional support were friends and teachers:

> "This amazing woman [her teacher], who is still a good friend of mine today, took me to a psychologist."

As far as the formal agents were concerned, most of the help-seekers consulted a professional therapist, but the consultation was not helpful. One obstacle in the path of an effective outcome of the professional therapy is the emotional difficulty that the disclosure of the traumatic experience entails. The medium of communication exerts a direct effect on the willingness to receive help:

> "I know about the emergency center for sexual abuse but I don't know if I can send them an email. I feel embarrassed to sit opposite a person and talk, and I can't do it over the phone."

Active coping: In two cases, the sexually-assaulted help-seekers reported the assault to the police. One of them went to the police with a friend, and the other went to the police with her mother shortly after the occurrence of the event. Theoretically, this active coping strategy is considered to be adequate in cases of traumatic events because it can help the victim regain a sense of control and possibly begin to repair her shattered self-confidence. In these two cases, however, the act of reporting the incident to others engendered negative consequences. In one case, both parents were judgmental instead of supportive, and in the other, the first encounter with the police was threatening, causing her to refuse to continue the formal complaint procedure:

> "I'm afraid they'll blame me for what happened. They'll say that it was my fault, that I shouldn't have gone to that place, that I didn't make any attempt to / fight back after he started."

She seemed to have found herself in a trap, since the recommended measures for coping with the trauma served merely to increase her distress. She was now forced to cope not only with the implications of the rape, but also with being a disappointment and a burden to the people close to her.

Appeal for online assistance: The analysis of the chats revealed that the decision to seek help via the personal chat stemmed from the combination of three factors: (1) the increasing desire to end the unbearable emotional distress; (2) the maturity to receive emotional assistance; and (3) viewing the anonymous personal chat as an appropriate communicative environment for appealing for assistance.

The desire to end the suffering is expressed explicitly in each of the chats:

> "I want to find ways to cope with the thoughts about it. I want to talk. I have to talk. Help me."
>
> "Once I asked for help and now I'm begging for help. I don't know what to do to get rid of it."

In the context of help-seeking, maturity is described both as a feeling of readiness to receive emotional assistance – a feeling that had not been experienced previously, and as a critical opportunity for change:

> "If I don't talk now, and indicate that I am ready for it now, I will simply go back a million steps, and I've already taken a step forward."

Further evidence of the readiness to receive assistance is found in the words of another help-seeker, who recounts her traumatic experience of the rape that occurred seven years prior to the chat. In order to actualize the potential readiness for assistance, the appropriate conditions are required; the personal chat is perceived as furnishing these conditions to a greater extent than alternative sources of assistance:

> "It is very uncomfortable for me to sit in front of a person and talk. It is also difficult to talk on the telephone."

"I've heard about the center for assisting sexually-assaulted women, but I don't know if I can talk to them online."

The help-seeker's first encounter with the volunteer was characterized by the former's hesitant and even apologetic approach:

"I'm sorry to bother you and maybe it's too much to ask, I'm sorry…"

"Hello, I don't know how this works, but I guess there are more important and more urgent things that you have to cope with. It's not urgent, I just need someone neutral to listen to me…perhaps a few pieces of advice, not more than that."

They construct the personal relationship with the volunteer slowly and gradually. One of them, for instance, positioned herself in relation to an abstract source of help:

"I need to talk and I'm begging for your help."

Another help-seeker attempted very hesitantly to obtain some information about the person on the other side of the chat:

"I know you're not allowed to give out personal details, but can you tell me if you are a man or a woman?"

The hesitant and cautious approach of the help-seekers with regard to seeking assistance from the chat probably resulted from the combination of several factors: the difficulty experienced by sexually-assaulted women to seek any type of assistance in which they will be required to reconstruct – and therefore re-experience – the traumatic event; the disappointment resulting from previous attempts to receive assistance; and the uncertain nature of the interaction in the personal chat. In spite of all these potential barriers, the victims actually took the first step in a continuous process of disclosing their experiences in an online environment. In all the chats that were analyzed, the process ended with expressions of gratitude to the volunteer as well as with indications of an effective outcome:

"Thank you for everything. You really helped me cope. I feel like I'm hurting less now."

"OK, I think I'll go back to preparing for my exam tomorrow."

"You have no idea how much you've helped me and what you've done for me."

Discussion

The present study set out to explore the unique value of the personal chat as a medium of communication for individuals suffering from anorexia and for individuals experiencing trauma resulting from sexual assault. These two types of help-seekers were chosen because of the emotional difficulty they experienced when seeking assistance from traditional face-to-face sources. We utilized transcripts of naturally-occurring personal chats in order to perform an in-depth observation regarding both their decision to seek assistance from the Internet and the nature of the assistance offered to them.

The analysis revealed that the decision to seek help via the chat was affected by processes that occurred in four different circles. The first circle focused on the help-seeker's psychological problem, particularly on the personal meaning she attributed to that problem. The second circle focused on the intra-personal aspect. The analysis of this circle revealed the help-seeker's perceptions with regard to herself – her characteristics, strengths, and weaknesses, beliefs concerning herself and her surroundings, and her desire to change her current condition. The third circle focused on the interpersonal aspect, and its analysis revealed how the help-seeker positioned herself in relation to figures in her environment such as family, friends, and therapists. The fourth circle emerged directly from the processes that occurred in the first three, which led to acute mental pain. This circle, which was constructed in order to stop the pain, is the coping circle. We shall present the characteristics of each circle as well as the processes that occur within each of them and among them, leading to the decision to seek assistance, and then evaluate the unique value of the personal chat for individuals who suffer from AN or from traumas resulting from sexual assault.

Perception of the problem: The present study focuses on two different psychological problems that share a common feature, namely, difficulty in seeking face-to-face assistance. From the psychiatric point of view, the two problems differ with regard to their symptomatology and etiology. They also differ in the course of their clinical development: while AN develops gradually, without a distinct onset, the traumatic reaction to sexual assault occurs abruptly as a result of an unexpected external event.

In spite of these clinical differences, the analysis of the chats revealed a striking similarity in the way the help-seekers described the implications of the problems for their well-being. Both the anorexia and the traumatic reaction were described as psychological entities with a strong, incessant presence in their lives, which seriously impaired their emotional well-being. The effect of the problem was evident in the emotional, cognitive, and behavioral realms. Emotionally, the help-seekers described prolonged periods of depression, anxiety, acute loneliness, and a loss of the will to live. Cognitively, they suffered from impaired self-esteem, severe self-criticism, and obsessive thoughts, all of which caused them to doubt their sanity. They were obsessed with thoughts of how they were perceived by their environment, and viewed themselves as a burden to their family and friends. Behaviorally, they reported a sharp decrease in the quality of performing everyday tasks in their studies or at work. The effect of their problem on their mental state can be summed up by the metaphors they employed in order to describe their lives: *"nightmare"*, *"life in the garbage"*, *"broken to pieces"*.

An additional characteristic that is common to AN and traumatic reaction following sexual assault is the psychological barrier that prevents the victims from seeking assistance. The chats with the individuals suffering from AN revealed a mechanism (which is inherent in the disorder) that inhibited their desire to seek professional therapy: they believed that the anorexia protected them by strengthening their self-control; consequently, they preferred to preserve this ability and view the therapy as an enemy. As regards the individuals who experienced sexual assault, their tendency to avoid seeking therapy resulted from the emotional threat associated with reconstructing – and therefore re-experiencing – the traumatic event. This threat was so powerful that they even eschewed calling a telephone help-line for victims of sexual assault because they would have to hear themselves uttering words such as "rape".

The findings of the present study, which demonstrate an attitude of hesitancy toward and avoidance of seeking emotional assistance, are consistent with the literature on individuals who suffer from AN (Goldner, Birmingham & Smye, 1997) and on individuals suffering from traumatic reaction following sexual assault (Campbell et al., 2001). It may be concluded that the psychological price associated with seeking assistance is higher than the potential benefits of receiving the assistance. The processes that drive the sufferer to stop the pain by seeking assistance occur in the same mental arena as the processes that inhibit her from appealing for assistance, thus engendering a help-seeking trap in which one hand reaches for assistance while the other strives to undermine this attempt.

Self-perception of the help-seeker: The discourse of the help-seekers revealed a difference in the characteristics of self-perception between individuals who suffered from AN and individuals who were victims of sexual assault. The adolescents and adult women suffering from AN described themselves using adjectives indicating an ongoing, stable self-perception that was not affected by a particular event:

> "I'm nothing, I'm garbage, I'm a statistical cipher."

It is reasonable to assume that their perception of themselves had been molded prior to the onset of the disorder and probably became more extreme as a result of their experience with it. The self-descriptions of the individuals who were sexually assaulted were directly related to the traumatic event. They described themselves as stressed, confused, worried, and guilty as a result of the event. Some of them even described a change that occurred between their present self-perception and their self-perception prior to the traumatic event:

> "I was a different person then. I changed so drastically."

However, the help-seekers in the two groups shared a common characteristic: they drew an absolutely negative self-portrait, which was firm and decisive. While there was no indication of a positive perspective, there was a dearth of personal resources, no hope, and not even a glimmer of optimism for the future. Their social identification was also painted in dark colors. They perceived themselves as alienated, rejected, hated (particularly the individuals suffering from AN), and ostracized by their surroundings (particularly those who had experienced sexual assault).

The implications of a self-perception of this kind can be destructive to the individual's mental and emotional well-being as well as to her social functioning. It drastically limits the space in which a productive, healthy life can be lived, and triggers mental pain that may become unbearable. This claim is corroborated by the desire to die, which was evident in the discourse of the help-seekers. A negative self-perception can affect mental health not only directly (as described above) but also indirectly, by impairing social relationships, as demonstrated in the interpersonal circle.

Interpersonal relationships: The most salient characteristic of the manner in which the help-seekers positioned themselves in relation to their social environment was alienation and disconnection. Their perception of the environment's attitude toward them constituted a dimension of alienation, with indifference at one end and repulsion at the other. They explained the source of the hostility of their environment toward them as residing in the burden that they were imposing on their immediate social setting, including the closest figures such as parents and friends. They invested a great deal of energy in concealing their mental condition in an attempt to protect their parents from the disappointment of having such a daughter, or to protect themselves from their parents' criticism and judgmental response. Their sense of alienation and rejection inevitably produced an acute feeling of loneliness. They were convinced that nobody could really understand the depth of their unique experience:

> "Nobody understands how it feels to be me and nobody shows any interest or tries to get into my heart."

The experience of social rejection prevented the individuals suffering from AN or from the trauma engendered by sexual assault from enjoying the benefits of the major resource for coping with loneliness and alienation, namely, social support. There is a huge body of knowledge demonstrating that social support is one of the most valuable and effective ways to cope with emotional distress. Social support constitutes a protective factor whose presence enhances emotional well-being and whose absence may create maladaptive reactions to stressful experiences (see Cohen & Wills, 1985; Sarason, Sarason & Pierce, 1990). The frustration resulting from the discrepancy between the need for social support and the failure to satisfy this need may lead to the espousal of alternative coping strategies. Such strategies are discussed in the following section.

Coping: The processes in the three circles mentioned above created a severe and ongoing stressful experience for the help-seekers. The problem itself – anorexia or traumatic reaction resulting from a sexual assault –exerted a direct effect on the individual's mental condition by producing symptoms of depression and anxiety. In addition, the problem had an indirect effect by shaping a negative, constricted, and devalued self-perception that intensified the anguish and impaired everyday functioning. The encounter between this type of self and the social environment did not generate an emotional connection and social affiliation, but rather led to acute loneliness and alienation. A stressful situation inevitably evokes the use of strategies that seek to end the tension and restore psychological equilibrium (Lazarus & Folkman, 1984) .

The analysis of the chats revealed that the online help-seekers employed a variety of strategies that can be categorized into two types according to their value in successful coping. The first type includes inadequate means of coping with the situations, such as an attempt to conceal the problem, self-harm, or avoidance of active coping. The second type includes strategies that are potentially helpful, such as seeking professional assistance. However, the encounter with the mental health professional did not lead to the desired outcome. In some cases, the therapy was helpful, but its effect was temporary. In other cases, therapeutic relationships did not develop due to mechanisms inherent in the problem itself, such as the need to preserve the symptoms (AN) or the emotional threat posed by self-disclosure (sexual assault). It is interesting to note that the coping strategies mentioned by the help-seekers did not include social support, which usually plays a vital role in coping with stressful experiences.

The discrepancy between continuous emotional distress and the lack of resources to cope with it successfully paved the way to the decision to seek assistance via the personal chat. While the help-seekers did not provide explicit reasons for choosing the chat, we can assume that this decision can be attributed to the unique features of the online environment that create the appropriate conditions for seeking help (Gilat & Shahar, 2009; Suler, 2004). The option to remain anonymous afforded the requisite emotional safety for self-disclosure, and the use of written texts as a channel of communication mitigated the threat of verbalizing traumatic experiences:

> "I can't say the word 'rape'."

In addition, the chat is more convenient – both practically and emotionally – than face-to-face communication. (For instance, if the client is disappointed, it is much easier to halt the chat than inform a therapist that she wants to terminate it.)

Coping by appealing for online assistance: The analysis of the online interactions with the individuals who suffered from AN or from the trauma engendered by sexual assault facilitated the identification of the unique processes that occurred during the chat and the evaluation of their contribution to the emotional welfare of the help-seekers. A major characteristic of these interactions, which was evident in all the chats that were analyzed, was the self-disclosure of the help-seekers. In their online encounter with the anonymous volunteers, they disclosed ultra-personal experiences, emotions, and thoughts, including the dark side of their selves. They explicitly expressed their self-hatred, their self-criticism, and their self-devaluation, which haunted their minds. They gave vent to the feelings of acute loneliness and social isolation that prevented them from establishing an emotional connection with their social surroundings and left them isolated and expendable. It appears that the online environment enabled them to overcome the barriers that had inhibited self-disclosure in their face-to-face communication with the agents of assistance to whom they had appealed prior to the chat.

Disclosing personal feelings and thoughts can be a liberating experience by reducing loneliness and producing social affiliation, as many studies have revealed, including studies that examined self-disclosure on the Internet (Bareket-Bojmel & Shahar, 2011; Boniel-Nissim & Barak, 2011). This liberating experience may be particularly significant among individuals suffering from AN or from the trauma resulting from sexual assault because not only do they avoid sharing their stressful experience with their environment, but they also expend a great deal of energy on concealing their situation and on broadcasting a message of “business as usual”. Since these efforts exact an emotional and functional price, the opportunity to disclose their feelings afforded by the online environment may be more helpful for them than for individuals suffering from problems such as depression and anxiety that cannot be concealed.

CONCLUSION

Individuals suffering from AN or from the trauma caused by sexual assault experience acute loneliness and social alienation, which jeopardize their emotional welfare and normal functioning. They avoid seeking professional assistance due to the need to preserve the symptoms (AN) or the threat associated with reconstructing the traumatic experience (sexual assault). Their eschewal of seeking professional assistance increases their distress and is liable to lead to suicidal thoughts. The personal chat with the trained volunteer creates an intimate, containing, and supportive environment in which they feel sufficiently safe to expose their real selves and experience an authentic encounter with another person, thereby constructing a bridge to the life of equilibrium that everyone craves.

The present chapter focused on individuals suffering from AN or from the trauma resulting from sexual assault and illuminated the unique value of the personal chats for them. We did not examine the characteristics of the volunteers' responses or their contribution to the outcome of the interactions with the help-seekers. This aspect constitutes the focus of the next chapter, in which we shall present empirical data regarding the benefit of personal chats to distressed individuals.

Chapter 5

RENDERING EMOTIONAL FIRST AID VIA EMAIL

ABSTRACT

Email constitutes one of the earliest online applications employed for rendering emotional first aid. The present chapter expounds the advantages and limitations of email as a mode of online assistance. It further presents empirical evidence regarding three aspects of the interaction between individuals who seek emotional first aid via email and ERAN's volunteers: (1) the domains of the problems presented by the help-seekers; (2) the type of assistance the help-seekers expect to receive; and (3) the response strategies employed by the volunteers in order to provide assistance. Finally, the advantages of email, the type of assistance, and the response strategies are exemplified in a case study of an interaction between a troubled adolescent and a trained volunteer.

INTRODUCTION

Letters were used for the purpose of rendering psychological assistance long before the Internet era. Freud, for instance, corresponded with his clients by letter, the most cited example thereof being the advice he gave to the father of "Little Hans" about dealing with his son (Freud, 1959). There were two advantages to communicating by letter in the pre-Internet period. First, the elimination of geographical barriers enabled the therapeutic process to continue when face-to-face contact was not feasible. Second, the use of letters liberated the two parties in the therapeutic encounter from the pressure of providing an immediate response and enabled them to plan their messages without being subjected to time pressure. In the Internet era, the use of electronic mail has expanded the range of advantages of letters as a channel of communication for providing psychological assistance since it exploits all the unique advantages of the online environment. This chapter presents the following aspects of rendering emotional first aid via email: (1) advantages and limitations of email as a source of assistance; (2) characteristics of the problems presented by individuals seeking emotional first aid via email; and (3) the strategies of assistance employed by the volunteers who respond to distressful messages.

Advantages of Assistance via Email

In order to gain an insight into the unique advantages of email as a source of emotional assistance, help-seekers who contacted ERAN via email were asked to explain why they had opted for this particular channel of communication. A content analysis of the responses yielded three advantages of this channel that can enhance the helpfulness of the help-seeking. The first is the use of writing for the purpose of communication. Writing was perceived as a convenient channel of communication since it gave the writer a sense of freedom from emotional barriers and permitted a more open and accurate expression of his/her feelings than oral discourse did:

> "I chose email because I'm ashamed to call the telephone help-line. I hardly use the telephone in my personal life and I prefer to use email."
>
> "It's much easier for me to talk about myself and to express my feelings in writing."
>
> "Writing gives me an opportunity to express myself accurately. Oral conversation inhibits me in my attempt to describe the problem as it is."

The second advantage of email is the pace of the communication. The time lapse between receiving and responding to the message affords the writer sufficient time to plan the message without the time pressure that exists in the personal chat. The writer can reread his/her original message and make the necessary alterations until it is satisfactory. While the possibility of planning the message is always valuable, it can be crucial in some situations – for instance, when the help-seeker feels that his/her problem is very complex, and it would be difficult to convey the full complexity in a real-time conversation.

Another situation is an initial appeal for assistance, accompanied by anxiety and inhibitions. The possibility of reading the entire message before pressing SEND offers emotional security. These advantages are illustrated in the responses of the individuals who turn to ERAN for assistance:

> "I felt deep down that I desperately needed someone to listen to me. I found the ERAN website on the Internet and saw that I could send an email. It's simpler than using the chat because it gives me time to formulate what I want to say. It's very difficult for me to express myself with regard to my problems, I've never tried to do it."
>
> "I felt that my story was long and complex and didn't suit the personal chat. With email it's easier to see in advance if I've succeeded in clarifying what I wanted to say."

The third advantage of email is the full documentation of the entire interaction. In face-to-face or oral conversation, the interaction is stored in the human memory and suffers from all the attendant biases. In contrast, the email interaction is documented and available to be read at any time:

> "[The volunteer's] responscs arc always long, with a great deal of investment and attention. In addition, I can always go back to the mail and read the response when I feel bad, when the chat is not available."
>
> "Your response enables me to read it slowly and understand the implications of my problem."

It is important to point out several limitations of therapy via email: (1) It is easy to misinterpret messages as a result of the absence of non-verbal cues; (2) The time-lag between the responses of therapist and client alike causes email therapy to be an inappropriate means of assistance in emergency situations that demand immediate intervention; (3) Unlike synchronous means of online communication – the personal chat, for instance – email interactions suffer from a lack of spontaneity; and (4) Emails may cause the client to over-analyze the therapist's responses.

The Content and Process of Emotional First Aid via Email

This section proffers empirical evidence pertaining to three aspects of the interaction between individuals who seek emotional first aid via email and ERAN's volunteers: (1) the domains of the problems presented by the help-seekers; (2) the type of assistance the help-seekers expect to receive; and (3) the response strategies employed by the volunteers in order to provide assistance. Data were gathered from 65 email interactions retrieved randomly from all the interactions that were recorded over a three-month period in 2011. The texts were analyzed by two mental health professionals who were experienced in online counseling. The analysis was conducted in keeping with the ground theory approach (Strauss & Corbin, 1990), according to which the categories are not predetermined by a theoretical framework, but rather emerge directly from the data.

Problem Domains

The analysis, which revealed a wide variety of problem domains presented by the distressful individuals who sought assistance via email, yielded ten categories of problem domains. Four of these categories relate to the interpersonal arena: loneliness, interpersonal relationships, marital relationships, parent–child relationships. Three categories represent types of psychological disorders: depression, anxiety, other mental disorders (see Table 1). Three categories relate to the environmental arena: school/work setting, military service, the security situation in Israel. Table 1 presents exemplary citations for each category. This variety of problem domains is consistent with the finding reported in Chapter 3, which is based on an independent sample of emails. The above-mentioned finding has encouraging implications for seeking psychological assistance since it shows that individuals in distress consider this unique source of assistance to be suitable for all types of problems. In light of the barriers involved in seeking face-to-face assistance, the attractiveness of the email expands the pool of available sources and the populations that can benefit from such assistance.

Table 1. Examples of problem domains presented by individuals seeking help from ERAN via email

Domain	Example
Depression	An 18-year-old girl describes her reaction to her friend's decision to end the relationship: *"I'm in total despair. I'm preoccupied with this all day long and my mood is so down since we separated (more than two months ago). I've lost my appetite and my grades have deteriorated and worst of all – my enjoyment of life has disappeared completely."*
Anxiety	A 25-year-old man discloses his feeling of anxiety, which occurred without any specific reason: *"I can't find words to describe what I'm experiencing. I'm inundated with anxieties and they are becoming more acute and more powerful. There are so many other things happening. I must find someone to talk to."*
Mental illness	A young woman describes dramatic changes in her sister's behavior: *"She has become very violent in the last weeks, mostly verbally. She loses control, fights with everyone for no reason, yells and shouts. I think she is going through a very severe crisis and she refuses to talk to a therapist. What should I do?"*
Marital problems	A man in his forties writes about a crisis in his marital life: *"We fight and fight every week or two. I feel that my marriage is coming to an end. I don't want it to end, but I'm tired of fighting. When I fight with her, I can't work and I can't smile and I become unbearable."*
Interpersonal relationships	A young man writes about his disappointment with people he met: *"I don't count on anyone in this world anymore. I've been disappointed by people too many times...I'm too hurt to share my feelings with people I see every day."*
Military service	A soldier in the infantry writes: *"I don't know what to do. I believe that if I stay in the army and obtain weapons, I'll do myself harm. I really, really don't know what to do with myself and I don't want to continue with my military service."*
Security situation	A girl who lives in an area that was attacked by missiles describes her feelings: *"I have anxieties, I keep seeing missiles, and when this happens again and again, I shake and shiver all over my body."*

Types of Expectations

The analysis of the email interactions yielded two types of expectations on the part of the help-seeker: problem-oriented and person-oriented. The first type is evidenced by the help-seeker's expectation of receiving assistance in the solution of a specific problem, for instance, how to cope with a sudden change in the behavior of the husband or how to choose between two equally attractive jobs. The second type is evidenced by the help-seeker's expectation of receiving assistance in eliminating an ongoing state of distress such as depression, anxiety, or the loss of a dear one, which undermines his/her sense of well-being. The common characteristic of these two patterns is the expectation of receiving instrumental assistance. Interestingly enough, the expectation of receiving emotional assistance such as social support, which is so prevalent in personal chats, was absent in the emails sent to ERAN.

Assistance Strategies

In the context of emotional first aid, an assistance strategy can be defined as a general pattern of response that is derived from a theoretical approach and whose objective is to offer psychological assistance to an individual in distress. The general pattern combines many specific responses, all of which emerge from the same approach and aim to achieve the same purpose. For instance, "providing emotional support" is a strategy that can be manifested in different responses that convey the same message of emotional support.

The analysis of the volunteers' responses to the individuals who sought assistance via email yielded three broad categories of strategies that were employed by the volunteers, and reflected three (not mutually exclusive) approaches to psychological assistance: emotion-oriented strategies, cognitive-oriented strategies, and behavior-oriented strategies.

The purpose of the *emotion-oriented approach* is to establish an emotional bond between the individual in distress and the help-giver. This emotional bond is critical in emotional assistance and constitutes an essential condition for achieving a successful outcome. The significance of the emotional bond stems from the very nature of human distress. In spite of both the variety of distress types and the subjective nature of the stressful experience, there is a common characteristic that can be defined as acute loneliness. Individuals who experience mental agony feel that they are unable to bear the heavy burden alone. The emotional connection offered by another person generates a feeling that he/she is not alone, increases his/her emotional well-being, and helps mobilize his/her internal resources for coping with the problem.

The *cognitive-oriented approach* seeks to effect a change in the meaning that the distressful person ascribes both to the situation and to him/herself. This change may be manifested in various components of the cognitive system such as beliefs, attitudes, expectations, and intentions. Unlike the emotion-oriented approach, which aims to achieve temporary relief in the help-seeker's emotional well-being, the cognitive-oriented approach aspires to create an enduring change in his/her system of beliefs – a change that will subsequently lead to an improvement in his/her emotional and behavioral systems. The desired goal of cognitive change can be accomplished in different ways such as offering the individual a more optimistic outlook on his/her situation, inspiring belief in the individual's ability to cope with the threatening situation, raising the individual's awareness of his/her internal and external resources, and suggesting unconventional ideas for solving the problem.

Table 2. Assistance strategies in the responses to help-seekers' emails

Approach	Strategy
Emotion-oriented	Conveying empathy
	Offering emotional support
	Self-disclosure of the help-giver
	Reflection
Cognitive-oriented	Reinforcing the decision to seek help
	Normalization
	Empowering the help-seeker
	Suggesting an alternative meaning
	Confrontation
	Providing constructive information
	Suggesting practical ideas
Behavior-oriented	Encouraging the help-seeker to seek further assistance

The *behavior-oriented approach* aims to help the individual effect a behavioral change such as reaching a decision or applying ideas in order to solve a problem. Since the boundaries differentiating among the three approaches are not clear-cut, some response strategies include components of more than one approach. For instance, the strategy of empowerment contains a clear cognitive component since its aim is to increase the individual's self-efficacy; however, it can also bring about an improvement in his/her emotional state. In order to present and illustrate the strategies employed by ERAN's volunteers in their email responses, each strategy has been classified according to one of the three approaches. The list of strategies is presented in Table 2, followed by clarifications and exemplifications.

Emotion-oriented Strategies

The strategy of *conveying empathy* is manifested in the help-giver's expression of understanding of the help-seeker's experience. Despite the fact that the word "understanding" derives from the semantic field of cognition, it is painted in emotional colors in the discourse of emotional first aid.

> "I understand that the environment in which you live is very unpleasant for you. It's probably an unbearable feeling to live in a place where people are so repulsive."
>
> "I understand your pain and your distressful feeling so well."
>
> "I'm not fully familiar with the feelings that you are experiencing, the pain, the depression, the lack of energy to do anything. But I can imagine how awful it is to live like that."

In face-to-face communication, messages of empathy can be conveyed not only verbally but also by means of eye contact, smiles, gestures, intonation, and physical contact. When communicating via email, the written language is the only medium for delivering emotional messages and establishing an emotional bond with the help-seeker. Therefore, the inclusion of direct, verbal, empathic messages in the email response is crucial.

The strategy of *emotional support* is manifested in the expression of positive feelings, which are directed at the individual in distress. Emotional support differs from empathy by dint of the personal involvement of the help-giver, who expresses his/her own feelings with respect to the help-seeker's emotional state.

> "I feel like giving you a big hug and helping you feel more relaxed."
>
> "I couldn't stop myself from sending you my deepest affection."

The strategy of *self-disclosure* is manifested in the volunteer's disclosure of a personal experience that is related to the help-seeker's emotional state. Self-disclosure can be effective in establishing an emotional bond with the help-seeker because it elicits in him/her a sense of solidarity and genuine understanding on the part of someone who is familiar with this feeling.

> "I know exactly what you're talking about because I've been there and I know that depression can drive you to places of despair and apathy. But believe me – it is possible to get out of there."

The strategy of *reflection* is manifested in the repetition of words, phrases, or sentences written by the help-seeker. In some cases, the help-giver uses the help-seeker's exact words, and in others, changes are made, but the reflection remains descriptive, without interpretation and without any effort to alter the meaning of what the help-seeker wrote. The reflection of emotional contents may help engender emotional relief in the help-seeker's state as a result of the very fact that another person is paying attention to him/her. The use of reflection is very convenient in email communication since the entire text sent by the help-seeker is available, and there is sufficient time to read it and decide on the elements to reflect.

> "You're very angry with yourself and the strong guilty feelings don't allow you to be calm."
>
> "There's something that only you know, something that you 'really' experience. There's the outside and there's the inside, and the distance between them seems so big right now."

Cognitive-oriented Strategies

The strategy of *reinforcing the decision to seek help* is manifested in attributing a positive significance to the very decision to seek emotional assistance. The use of this strategy is particularly important when the help-seeker manifests hesitation and doubt regarding help-seeking and tends to perceive it as a weakness. By suggesting that the help-seeking be viewed as proof of strength rather than as a sign of weakness, we help the help-seeker develop a more positive attitude both toward seeking help and toward him/herself. Moreover, this positive attitude can increase the help-seeker's willingness to take responsibility during the therapeutic process, thereby achieving a more effective outcome.

> "Thank you for choosing to write this email. I think you're very brave. The fact that you are seeking assistance is a source of power."

The strategy of *normalization* is manifested in changing the meaning of seeking assistance from an unusual, abnormal phenomenon into a normative situation that is quite prevalent among the general population. Viewing the threatening situation as normative may help the troubled individual when he/she labels him/herself “different”, “odd”, or “wacko”, and consequently eschews seeking assistance. Moreover, the belief that the problem is unique magnifies the subjective threat as well as the fear that nobody could possibly understand him/her and rescue him/her from it. In online support groups, normalization is achieved by means of the group process, during which the individual reaches the realization that he/she is not alone. In email assistance, normalization is achieved by means of the message sent to the help-seeker by the volunteer.

> “Feelings like those you describe are very common among adolescents.”
>
> “First of all, I can assure you that such feelings of 'down' are normal and natural among people of your age.”

The strategy of *empowerment* is manifested in raising the help-seeker's awareness of his/her innate personal resources. The latter may include traits, abilities, skills, beliefs, and achievements. Empowerment can be particularly effective if the personal resources mentioned by the help-giver are based on the interaction itself.

> “Your language is so rich and beautiful, your analysis of yourself and your insights is so intelligent.”
>
> “You are a person who really wants and looks for a change in his life. You don't give up, don't run away, but you dare to do things.”

The strategy of *suggesting an alternative meaning* aims to transform the threatening or pessimistic meaning that the help-seeker ascribes to an event, to a certain type of behavior, or to himself, into a more encouraging meaning.

In response to a message from a man who had lost his wife and wrote that he had joined an online dating service, a volunteer wrote:

> “What you did is not what you think it is, but rather the initiative of a healthy man who wants to get on with his life in spite of the pain.”

In response to a teenager who described his father's authoritarian behavior, a volunteer wrote:

> "You wrote that your father sets strict limits. Let's look at it from a different angle. Your father probably loves you very much, cares about you, and worries because you are so important to him. You are probably aware of the outbreak of violence in the streets nowadays. Parents naturally want to protect their children."

In the strategy of *confrontation*, the responder confronts the help-seeker with the dangerous implications of a certain idea or type of behavior for his/her welfare. The natural tendency of people to preserve the existing system of beliefs and behavior prevents them from realizing the hazardous consequences of this system. The strategy of confrontation aims to reassess the existing beliefs.

In response to a father who described conflicts with his adolescent daughter, a volunteer wrote:

> "The more responsibility you take for your daughter's tasks, the less responsibility she will take. I've no doubt that your intentions are good, but the result is that the child knows that someone will always 'rescue' her from any difficulty and she won't make any effort of her own."

Behavior-oriented Strategies

The strategy of *suggesting practical ideas* aims to furnish the help-seeker with practical ideas that may help him/her take the necessary steps to solve a problem. The issue of advice-giving is controversial in the domain of psychological assistance. One approach posits that the help-giver should avoid giving advice because it may trigger a dependent attitude on the part of the help-seeker and prevent him/her from assuming personal responsibility and making independent decisions. Advice pertaining to cardinal areas of the help-seeker's life, such as marriage or career planning, is particularly dangerous since the price for erroneous advice may be very high. Conversely, another approach states that advice can be very helpful owing to the help-givers' knowledge, experience, and ability to observe the situation from a rational perspective without emotional involvement. In addition, help-seekers should be given credit for their ability to make their own decision even when they request advice.

The analysis of the volunteers' responses revealed that while they did not refrain from giving advice, it was chosen carefully and did not entail a serious risk for the help-seekers.

"What do you think of inviting your mother to a personal conversation, explaining that you have something important you want to tell her privately? From the way you write, I believe that you would be able to disclose your feelings and simply tell her how you feel."

The strategy of *encouraging the help-seeker to seek additional assistance* is manifested in encouraging the help-seeker to seek additional social support in order to better cope with the problem and increase his/her emotional welfare. The use of this strategy is based on the knowledge of the helpfulness of social support on the one hand, and the high availability of sources of support on the other. These sources can be informal figures in the close environment of the help-seeker, para-professional agencies, or professional therapists.

"This change is difficult to make all alone. It will be much easier for you if you share it with someone close to you."

A Case Study of a Response via Email

The email presented and analyzed in this section was written by a volunteer in response to an email received from a 16-year-old girl. The latter presented herself as "an ordinary girl" who had undergone dramatic changes in her mood and in her everyday behavior during the previous two months. She felt very depressed, was troubled by anxiety, shunned participating in everyday activities, did not attend school (although she was an excellent pupil), and suffered from a lack of energy. This mental condition, which was unfamiliar to her and which persisted for several weeks, provoked thoughts and caused her to wonder:

"Am I really thinking about suicide? Looking for ways? Is this depression normal?"

For ethical reasons, we have not reproduced the girl's entire email; nevertheless, her messages can be easily deduced from the volunteer's response, which is presented with comments regarding the response strategies and their significance.

> "Hello my dear.
> Before writing anything, I want to thank you for writing this email to ERAN, for placing your trust in us, and for telling us so frankly and clearly what you have been through during the last months. A person, especially a young one, requires a great deal of mental strength to decide to sit down and write about such feelings and bad moods."

The volunteer employed two strategies in this opening passage, namely, (1) *reinforcement of the appeal for assistance* –the volunteer's legitimation of the very act of appealing for assistance is significant in view of the doubts and the self-blame conveyed by the girl with respect to her appeal for help:

> "I feel ridiculous for writing you this email",

and (2) *empowerment* – the volunteer stressed the abilities and strengths that came to the fore in the girl's email. Perhaps the decision to begin the response by reinforcing the appeal for help and empowering the help-seeker was based on the possibility that it would engender a positive attitude on the part of the girl toward the volunteer. This type of stance was necessary if the volunteer planned to effect a cognitive change and suggest an alternative outlook with regard to the girl's ostensibly unsolvable situation. The girl would probably be more attentive to a cognitive message once she perceived the sender as a supporter. In therapeutic terms, this phase is similar to creating a "therapeutic alliance", which depicts the therapist as friendly, caring, and committed.

> "I have read your email thoroughly several times and I want to tell you that I am greatly impressed with your ability to express yourself, with the richness and the clarity of your messages by means of which you have succeeded so well in conveying your bad feelings. You have experienced severe distress in the last couple of months and I understand you so much. You may not be surprised to hear that you are not alone. First of all, I am here with you, and second, these moods of depression and the feeling that there's no reason to get up in the morning are prevalent among teenagers."

In addition to the strategy of empowerment employed at the beginning of this passage, the volunteer implemented two additional strategies, namely, (1) *emotional support*, which was transmitted by expressions of understanding and by the promise, *"I am here with you"*, and (2) *normalization* – the volunteer suggested a normative meaning for the girl's severe emotional state, claiming her condition to be prevalent among adolescents. This approach may reduce anxiety in light of the fact that adolescents tend to view their problems as extremely severe and unique, and consequently unsolvable.

> "As I've already told you, you express your bad feeling so well: 'I'm beginning to decline in everything… my grades, my social status, my family, my functioning, and mainly myself. I feel that I'm beginning to lose my mind, and the truth is that it's very difficult for me because it exists and it's real more than ever, but I don't want to accept it.' Yes, my dear, this feeling is very scary because it depicts your entire current existence as senseless and meaningless and worst of all – it leaves no room for positive thinking. It's a new and strange feeling and it's natural that you refuse to accept it, because why did it invade your life all of a sudden and upset your whole world?! I know it's very painful and very frightening. The good news is that you are not alone in these thoughts. Feelings such as those you describe are very common among adolescents, as I've told you. But the fact that all these feelings and thoughts and distress are common among youngsters does not improve your mood, nor do they help you with your bad mood in the morning and low motivation to get up and go to school. It's quite obvious, and we'll return to this point later."

In this passage, the volunteer employed the strategy of reflection by repeating what the girl wrote and also by summarizing the girl's condition. Besides reflection, the volunteer also delivered empathic messages and suggested that the girl view her stressful situation as normative. The aim of the increased use of these strategies was to establish a positive emotional climate as well as trust in the volunteer, and also to trigger changes in the girl's perception of herself and her situation.

> "I understand that you have two good friends with whom you are sharing your experience, indicating that you are a sociable person who trusts whom she chooses to trust and knows how to disclose her feelings, which is, of course, very important. No one is a lone island in the stream of life, but the fulfillment of your emotional needs through the support and empathy of your friends is not enough, and in response to your important question, 'What am I supposed to do?', I am allowing myself to suggest a few other things: Make every effort to talk to your mother and share with her, even a little, what you feel and what you are going through. Your mother only sees your overt behavior, what can be seen from the outside – for instance, that you don't wake up by yourself, that you're late for school, that you go to school and come back an hour later, and so on. You yourself said that no one in the world, except your two good friends, has any idea of what you really feel.

> Not even your mother. What do you think about making an effort to talk to your mother about your feelings? Invite her to a neutral place and tell her whatever you choose to tell. Your mother may become the most devoted partner if you only let her."

In this passage, the volunteer employed a behavior-oriented strategy and advised the girl to disclose her inner pain and bewilderment to her mother. It is interesting to note how the volunteer constructed this part of the response. She began with an empowering comment about the girl's ability to share her feelings with others (her friends) and continued with the suggestion that she share her feelings with her mother. This advice could be very useful in view of the fact that the mother was unaware of the severity of her daughter's suffering. On the other hand, the girl did not provide information regarding her relationship with her mother. A state of tension might exist between the mother and her teenage daughter, and in this case, the volunteer's advice would not be useful.

> "And obviously, my dear, it can be helpful to seek assistance from a professional. When our body hurts, we go to an expert physician, and when the mind hurts, it's natural to seek assistance from an expert in the mind. Good friends are a valuable asset. They can reflect us ourselves, they can illuminate hidden areas in our selves, make us happy. But in many cases, this is not sufficient, and a skilled professional is required.
>
> Before I finish my response, I would like to copy a sentence that you wrote (and I'm taking it out of its original context) – '...and I do want to find one reason in order to show myself that I have something to live for, to prove to myself that I am wrong and that I do want to live...' – and ask you to read this sentence again in this optimistic context. It's your sentence, you wrote it yourself, and it contains powers of life and good energies. Don't ignore it! Even though there are moments, or weeks or months (and each one of us goes through such periods) when everything seems meaningless and you hear loud sounds of distress – you can overcome it, and with appropriate professional assistance, the sky will become clear and the sounds of life will win. And you have those strengths, they are self-evident."

In this passage, the volunteer illuminated the positive aspect of the distressful context within which the girl described her condition. This positive perspective is based on a quotation from the girl's email, thus increasing its validity. This passage – which may be viewed as a phase in an interactive process – focuses on inducing a cognitive change. The volunteer suggested that the girl change her interpretation of her inner turmoil and discover a source of strength and hope:

> "You do not seem to me to be a girl who is frustrated with life. You seem to be an intelligent girl who is facing a dramatic change in her attitude toward life, a change that is new and strange to her, scares her, threatens her, and drives her to behaviors that provoke conflicts with her environment. As you cope with this hurtful situation, you, like many other adolescents, even arrive at thoughts about suicide. The trouble with suicide is that it is not reversible. And I'd very much like to write a sentence that I've been debating with myself whether or not to do so since the beginning of this response, but I feel close enough to you, so I'm going to dare to say it: Don't waste your life. It is a gift that each of us has received, and each of us has a certain purpose here. I believe that with all my heart. You, too, have a purpose! I'm sure you have hobbies, things you love to do such as playing, singing, drawing, raising animals, traveling, perhaps doing something good for other people such as children with special needs. Do you have a community involvement program at school? The fun and the satisfaction from doing something good for others, even something small, are enormous."

The volunteer did not shy away from coming to grips with the suicidal aspect that was implicit in the email sent by the girl. She decided to raise this issue towards the end of the reply, after – hopefully – inspiring in the girl a positive attitude toward her. The arguments she raised concerning the suicidal thoughts might have been perceived as a cliché had they been conveyed at an earlier stage of the response. And yet she employed a sophisticated method to create intimacy – she shared her hesitations regarding delivering this message with the girl:

> "And I'd very much like to write a sentence that I've been debating with myself whether or not to do so since the beginning of this response, but I feel close enough to you, so I'm going to dare to say it."

She began with general message about the meaning of life and then applied the suicide message to the girl's personal characteristics and resources that emerged earlier in her email.

> "You know, I'm sitting here, writing you this email and trying to imagine how you'll react when you read my messages. I pray that my words find a path to your heart. I want to thank you again for your sharing and openness,

> [and I] wish you much enjoyment of youth in the times to come, with spring blooming in nature and in your heart."

In this final passage of the response, the volunteer chose to express her personal sense of caring. A message of this type may be powerful in view of the attitude of trust that was probably being established throughout the response. This final message provides closure since the email assistance provided by ERAN is defined as a single session: the help-seekers are not invited to respond, and most of them in fact do not send a response. In some cases, however, they choose to do so. The troubled girl presented in this case study is an example of a help-seeker who sent a response a few days after receiving the volunteer's email.

> "Hello, I received your email and read it so many times, and if we are talking about quoting – 'I am sitting here trying to imagine...' – the tears came back to my eyes because of these words. This horrible period that I'm trying to stop with each day that passes, I've decided to end by forcing myself to do it, by repression, or it may just pass because I've had enough.
>
> After that frightening day, I decided to begin studying more seriously, and I actually prepared for a test I have today and hope to pass. I believe that the behavior I told you about was exaggerated, and I have a feeling that I made a bit of a mess of things. Some of the teachers have told me that they want to talk to me, and I think it's about my grades, which have decreased sharply, and also about my inattentiveness in their lessons. The first meeting is tomorrow morning.
>
> As for my mother I don't intend telling her anything. I know that after I spent two whole days in my room, she feels alienated from me, and it's also because of my attitude toward her. As for the psychologist, I decided to go by myself. I don't know what will come of it, but maybe it's the right thing to do.
>
> So I'll end this email with many thanks, thank you very much. You deserve thanks because you cared about me. It made a big difference, I assure you. It hasn't caused a drastic improvement, but it's something that made me feel much better, so thank you.☺"

This case study illustrates the unique merits of emotional first aid in general and the medium of email in particular as sources of psychological assistance for individuals in distress. The girl who sent the email had no history of psychiatric or psychological disorders (as far as can be deduced from her message), and she had probably not sought psychological assistance from a formal source previously. In mid-adolescence, she realized that she was facing a stressful experience reminiscent of the well-known "storm and stress" concept proposed by Stanley Hall (Larson & Ham, 1993), which unsettled and worried her, and even induced her to entertain suicidal thoughts. There was an urgent need for psychological assistance. Where could she find an appropriate source of assistance? A professional therapist might be perceived as too threatening in view of her normative background. She did not even hint at this option in her mail.

Informal sources were also inappropriate: she viewed her mother as a source of stress rather than as an agent of emotional support; her adolescent friends were probably preoccupied with their own troubles, besides lacking the requisite experience and perspective that only an adult can offer in order to provide meaningful support for an individual in crisis. Volunteer-based emotional first aid can meet the needs of girls like this who are seeking assistance. The option to remain anonymous affords the emotional safety required for self-disclosure. The use of volunteers has two advantages: on the one hand, it minimizes the stigma that may be associated with the decision to seek help, and on the other, it provides help-seekers with assistance from semi-professionals.

The reasons for choosing to write an email out of all the available channels of assistance offered by ERAN, which include, besides email, a telephone hotline, a personal chat, and an online support group, are not explicitly stated by the girl, but can be surmised. One reason is the preference for writing as a mode of communication, which can be deduced from the quality of her writing: the email is well-written and well-organized, the language is rich (far superior to that of the average Israeli adolescent), and the entire message is clear and convincing. Perhaps a second reason is the preference for asynchronous communication, which gives the help-seeker a sense of freedom because he/she is not obliged to become involved in an interpersonal synchronous interaction.

The reasons mentioned above are consistent with the findings of a recent study (Gilat & Reshef, in press) in which help-seekers who utilized ERAN's email service were requested to give their reasons for selecting this particular medium. The findings revealed the most widespread reason for choosing email to be the fact that the help-seekers preferred writing as a means of communication. The second most widespread reason was the availability and accessibility of receiving help. Additional reasons were anonymity and asynchronous communication, since the latter affords the requisite amount of time for the proper presentation of the problem.

CONCLUSION

The use of email for emotional first aid is not simply an expansion of the repertoire of services available to troubled individuals in search of emotional assistance. Email has unique features that render it particularly suitable for individuals who may not feel comfortable with other sources. The unique value of email – for help-seekers and responders alike – stems from the combination of asynchronous communication and the use of writing as a means of communication. Help-seekers can convey their messages in a detailed, clear, and well-organized fashion. Besides this cognitive advantage, the fact that they can describe the details of their experiences in writing may also afford them emotional relief. Similarly, the responders have sufficient time to plan their responses (and to consult with others, if necessary). Furthermore, the help-seekers' messages are available as sources of reference in their entirety when the help-givers respond (e.g., quoting, reflecting, and referring to each subject broached by the help-seeker). Interestingly enough, these advantages already existed in the old version of email –letters – but the features of the online environment have upgraded the use of email and transformed it into a unique and valuable source for rendering emotional assistance.

Chapter 6

Online Support Groups

Abstract

The social support afforded members of a group within the context of the online environment constitutes the essence of one of the major sources of emotional support in the 21st century. This chapter presents the theoretical background of the three components of the phenomenon: social support, therapeutic value of group processes, and online environment. Both the advantages of online support groups and their limitations are described. Empirical evidence pertaining to the helpfulness of online support groups is presented, and the effect of an online support group moderated by trained volunteers is illustrated via an analysis of an entire thread retrieved from the online support group operated by the Israeli Association for Emotional First Aid (ERAN).

Introduction

From the very inception of the Internet, group-communication technologies were implemented in order to render emotional assistance. The first instances of online assistance in a group environment took the form of expert consultation and self-aid groups (Stoney, 1998). Subsequently, support groups moderated by professionals or trained volunteers became available to the surfers. Within a short period, online support groups had become an extremely popular mode of emotional assistance; today they constitute a valuable source of assistance within the repertoire of mental health agencies. The most widely-used technology for the online support group is the forum, namely, an electronic notice-board that is displayed when an individual enters a website. Every participant in the forum can send a message (or "post") to the board or a response to messages posted by others. The unit of interaction, which includes the opening post and subsequent responses, is known as a "thread". The communication is asynchronous, that is, the responses are subject to a time delay rather than dispatched immediately. While the duration of the delay varies, it usually ranges from a few minutes to several hours. Participation in the forum can be active (participants send posts), or passive (participants read the texts without intervening – this is known as "lurking").

The phenomenon of the online support group comprises three theoretical domains: social support, group processes, and online communication. Social support is regarded as one of the most significant means of rendering troubled individuals emotional assistance. Although there are various methods whereby social support can be provided, they all share the same objective: to empower the person in distress and prevent further deterioration in crisis situations. Theory, research, and practice have shown group processes to be powerful instruments that affect the emotional reactions and attitudes of the individuals who take part in them.

The online environment possesses communicative features that can increase the efficacy of emotional assistance. The combination of the power of the group and the enhancement of the therapeutic atmosphere in the online environment may be a powerful vehicle for coping with ongoing distress, as illustrated in the following post that was sent to the online support group operated by ERAN:

> "When I first joined the forum, I had already decided to commit suicide. I was so amazed by the warmth and the many responses I received that I put this intention aside. It still exists, but a moment before I decide, I enter the forum. I receive so much support and I realize that I should call my therapist." (Gilat, 2008).

Social Support

Social support is considered to be a phenomenon pertaining to interpersonal interaction, comprising one or more of the following components: emotional bonds, social reassurance, sharing information, and instrumental assistance (Caplan, 1974). This view implies a direct link between social support and the emotional well-being of the individual. Indeed, the professional literature furnishes evidence of the helpful effect of social support in promoting social adjustment and in coping with stress and crisis (Sarason, Sarason & Pierce, 1990).

Theoretically, the significance of social support can be explained by the role it plays in satisfying the individual's basic needs, particularly affiliation and being loved by significant figures. The theory of attachment (Bowlby, 1969) posits that emotional support and caring on the part of significant figures are essential conditions for the development of self-esteem and for the establishment of healthy interpersonal relationships. The need for emotional support does not disappear as an infant grows, but rather is manifested in a different form. The unidirectional pattern of dependence on the social environment changes to interdependence, in which the individual needs support from the environment but at the same time also supports others.

Another theoretical perspective regarding the value of social support stresses the three types of benefit that the individual can derive from it: emotional, cognitive, and behavioral. Emotionally, support from the environment engenders a sense of security by creating a bond with others and conveying the message to the individual that he/she is not alone in coping with stress and crisis. The cognitive contribution is evidenced by supplying useful information and empowering the individual's internal resources. Behaviorally, social support is manifested in practical ideas for coping with problems.

Two models have been proposed in order to explain the process whereby social support is related to emotional well-being. The model of indirect influence asserts that social support exerts a buffering effect on stress since it acts as a barrier against the dangerous implications of stressful experiences. Consequently, individuals who live in a supportive environment cope better with stressful events than individuals who lack support and are more vulnerable. According to this model, social support affects the well-being of the individual only in situations of stress and crisis.

The second model claims that social support exerts a direct effect on well-being – an effect that is positive and not limited to stressful events. This model asserts that social support is a basic human need whose absence impairs the individual's mental health and whose presence enhances it. Numerous studies on the effect of social support demonstrate both patterns of influence on well-being. (For a detailed review, see Cohen & Wills, 1985.)

One of the most commonly-used means of applying the idea of social support to real life is the self-aid group. While it is likely that people have always given support in informal contexts, formal groups only began to operate in the first half of the 20th century with the establishment of Alcoholics

Anonymous. The latter was a group framework for individuals suffering from alcohol addiction who conducted their encounters on the basis of several guidelines, namely, sharing mutual experiences, avoiding judgmental responses, and encouraging changes in the undesirable behavior. The number of self-aid groups has proliferated rapidly since the 1980s, and today they are regarded as one of the major sources of social support.

In spite of the variations in the nature of support groups, there are several characteristics that are common to most of them. *The purpose* of the group is to afford the participants social support. This support is transmitted via a process in which all the members share their feelings, thoughts, and dilemmas, and receive feedback and responses from the other members of the group. These responses include emotional expressions of support such as empathic understanding, direct affection, and emotional bonding by sharing their own experiences with the problem. *The members* of the group are all characterized by the fact that they are grappling with a similar type of problem such as a medical condition, psychological disorder, or tragic circumstances. As regards *leading the group*, in most cases the participants share the responsibility for the interactions, and the moderator's role is to direct the processes while going along with the members' preferences. In some cases, there is no formal moderator; in others, the role of moderator rotates among the members; and in still others, there is an external moderator.

Support groups differ from therapeutic groups in most characteristics: the purpose of therapeutic groups is to effect enduring changes in the participants' self-perceptions or patterns of behavior; the moderator is a mental health professional; and the setting of the group (number of participants, number of meetings) is more structured than that of support groups. Online support groups can be considered the electronic version of the traditional face-to-face self-aid groups. They have adopted the rationale and the guiding principles of the traditional groups, but they are conducted in the online environment, which affords them some advantages in achieving their purpose. The next section presents the characteristics of online support groups and their role in enhancing the helpfulness of this medium.

Advantages of Online Support Groups

The features of the online environment that increase openness and self-disclosure were described in detail in Chapter 2. To recapitulate, online support groups possess two salient features that increase the members' willingness to disclose their feelings and experiences. First, the option to remain anonymous provides the requisite emotional safety for self-disclosure since the group member is liberated from the anxiety associated with what others would think of him/her if they knew his/her problems. Second, the fact that the participants neither see nor hear one another nullifies status differences and obviates the fear of authority, thereby enabling them to express what they really think and feel. Self-disclosure is particularly important in support groups since the principal condition for the effectiveness of such groups is the members' willingness to reveal their authentic selves to the group. If a member shares his/her deepest and most personal experiences with the group, the other members can form an emotional bond and provide meaningful emotional support. Furthermore, the assistance offered by the other members may be more helpful if the full dimensions of the problem are disclosed. Typical evidence of the enhancing effect of self-disclosure was found in a study examining an online support group for individuals suffering from dental anxiety (Buchanan & Coulson, 2007). The participants attributed the effectiveness of the intervention to the nature of the communication in the group, which inspired them with the confidence to disclose their fears. Prior to joining the group, they had refrained from talking about their dental anxieties in order to avoid other people's judgmental reaction. They reported that as a result of the atmosphere in the online support group that encouraged members to be themselves, they had already experienced a sense of release from their fears during the earliest phase of the interaction.

Another example of the significance of the liberating atmosphere in the group was reported by Gilat and Rosenau (2004), who investigated the online support group operated by ERAN. They describe the case of an adolescent boy who disclosed his suicidal ideations and philosophical thoughts about life and death. At the beginning of the post, he wrote that he had mustered the courage to send the message only because he could remain anonymous. The two examples presented above attest to the unique significance of the online support group, namely, that the participants in these studies would have not sought any form of face-to-face assistance.

Eliminating Time Barriers: Emotional Assistance is Always Available

Technologically, the online support group can be conducted in a chat room, where the participants determine the time of the encounter in advance, and communication occurs in real time. In practice, this type of support group is rare, and the vast majority of online support groups utilize asynchronous communication, meaning that the responses are sent with a time delay. The potential advantages of asynchronous communication are unique to the online environment and can be beneficial to the individual who is seeking support, for the responders who are offering the support, and for the group process. The benefit to the sender of the message is the emotional relief gained from the mere act of writing down personal experiences. Even if the writer does not receive immediate feedback, writing can be a relieving and even a therapeutic experience (Boniel-Nissim & Barak, 2011). Thus, if a group member feels acute loneliness at three a.m., he/she can write down his/her feelings and send the message to the forum, knowing that it will be received by a supportive environment. As regards the responder, the asynchronous nature of the interaction obviates the need for an immediate response, which is characteristic of synchronous means of communication such as the personal chat, and permits the responder to reread the message, plan the response, write it as clearly as possible, and even consult someone prior to sending it.

Eliminating Geographical Barriers

The communication in online support groups completely eliminates barriers of geographical distance, thereby fulfilling Marshall McLuhan's vision of “the Global Village” (1964). This feature grants online support groups two advantages that face-to-face support groups lack. First, individuals with limited mobility due to physical, geographical, or other constraints also have the possibility of participating in the group. Online support groups constitute the sole opportunity for these individuals – who, in many cases, are in greater need of emotional support than others – to receive such support. Second, the “global village” atmosphere creates a sense of human solidarity that fosters intimacy, understanding, and supportive behavior.

Using Written Texts

The effect of writing in order to enhance self-disclosure and increase emotional well-being is evidenced by all online applications such as the personal chat, email, and the forum. However, there are unique advantages to the use of written texts in the online support group. One interesting phenomenon of writing in the online group is the variety of genres employed by the participants. These genres range from speech-like writing, which is characteristic of the personal chat, to the traditional writing that can be found in web pages. For instance, a single thread may contain a dialogue between two participants that resembles spontaneous speech on the one hand, and a long, well-organized message that resembles a traditional piece of writing on the other.

The unique characteristics of the forum permit the participants to utilize various types of writing, creating a blend of genres within the same environment. Participants can choose the genre that best suits them. An interesting example is the use of poetic writing that is embedded in the text of a thread. Following is an interaction from the ERAN forum, in which a group member in distress and a trained volunteer exchanged poems:

The message:

"Just not hugs
It does not help, it hurts.
A hug is not a present,
It is a transaction,
A hug comes with an obligation–
an obligation for affection,
an obligation to give back a hug,
an obligation that the hug will help."

The response:

"I would like to embrace you with a hug,
A hug that is entirely tenderness,
To walk with you hand in hand
To a land, where a man to a man is a brother.
I would like to carry you in my arms,
And offer you my heart as a place of serenity."

The Therapeutic Power of Group Processes

Social support afforded by a group is more powerful than the support offered in a personal situation because the group processes seem to exert an empowering effect on the participants. These group processes were investigated extensively by Yalom (1970), who identified several processes and characterized their effect on the group participants. Yalom's analysis was based on the face-to-face group, but subsequent studies revealed that the processes also occur in online groups (Barak, Boniel-Nissim & Suler, 2008; Weinberg, Uken, Schmale &Adamek, 1995). Four such processes are described below.

1. *Universality* is evidenced by the recognition that other people also have problems similar to yours. This recognition encourages group members to reveal their inner selves since they feel that the other members can understand them better because of the shared experience.
2. *Group cohesion* occurs when the awareness of the mutual experience creates emotional bonds among the members of the group. The cohesion is evidenced by group norms that encourage and even reward openness and self-disclosure. Group cohesion is considered to be a powerful aspect of the group dynamics because it generates a sense of belonging and sparks commitment on the part of the other members.
3. *Altruism* is manifested in expressions of caring and genuine concern for other group members. Altruism exerts a positive effect on both parties in the interaction. A person toward whom a caring and supportive attitude is expressed feels loved, worthy, and affiliated. A person who engages in altruistic behavior feels satisfied and rewarded by the act of giving.
4. *Inspiring hope* means the engendering of an optimistic attitude toward the future.

The effect of the group processes on the well-being of the individual members can be exemplified by an event that took place in the online support group operated by ERAN. A 17-year-old boy sent a message announcing that it was his birthday in five days' time and stating that he was expecting a very miserable birthday because he knew that no one would come. One of the group members organized a "surprise party", and on the boy's birthday, a beautifully designed post containing good wishes from other members was posted. The boy responded that never in his life had he felt so excited.

Types of Assistance Offered by Online Support Groups

While some online support groups offer general assistance in any problem domain, most of the groups concentrate on a specific domain and invite individuals who are grappling with a specific problem to join them. The variety of problems dealt with by online support groups is enormous, as can be learned from perusing lists of groups operating on the Internet. In spite of the variety of domains, the online support groups are rather similar in terms of their purposes and group processes (as described in the previous section). Is the type of assistance received by the participants specific – in other words, does it depend on the domain of the group? Or is it general – in other words, does it depend on the group processes? The literature on support groups describes two approaches regarding the types of assistance.

The first approach is illustrated in the article written by Barak, Boniel-Nissim, and Suler (2008), in which the authors analyzed the type of assistance offered in many online support groups and concluded that participation in the group does not lead to changes in specific domains but rather to a general improvement in the participants' emotional well-being. For instance, a support group for the alcohol-addicted does not cure the addiction, nor does a group for individuals suffering from depression lower the level of depression. The above-mentioned authors contend that the assistance received by the members in these two groups and in other groups that focus on a specific domain takes the form of the empowerment of the participants. This is manifested in improved general emotional well-being, increased self-efficacy and self-control, diminished feelings of loneliness, and the espousal of a more optimistic outlook. Empowerment increases the participants' ability to cope with stressful situations regardless of the type of stress.

The second approach contends that participation in online support groups can lead to a specific change in the problem that is shared by the participants in a specific group. Three examples of specific assistance are presented in the next section.

Processing the Experience of Loss

The loss of a significant person undermines the individual's psychological equilibrium and triggers the need to process the distressing experience. The processing of loss, known as the "mourning process", is necessary in order to gradually restore mental equilibrium and enable the individual to adjust to the new reality. Mourning is manifested in three modes: personal, interpersonal, and social. A major component of this process is sharing feelings and thoughts with others and receiving emotional and instrumental support from the environment. In some cases, it is difficult for people to go through the mourning process and they try to forego it and resume their normal routine too abruptly. If they eschew the normal process of mourning, they might pay a psychological price by fixating on the mourning and not attempting to restore their equilibrium.

The above-mentioned problem is liable to arise in the case of the suicide of a loved one. Suicide is often associated with feelings of guilt and shame on the part of the family, who, in consequence, attempt to conceal the circumstances of the death and avoid discussing the event and their experience with their social environment. The tension between the natural need to share their feelings with others on the one hand and refraining from doing so on the other might induce a serious impairment in their well-being and social functioning. Theoretically, an online support group can serve as a suitable environment for family members whose loved one committed suicide.

The claim mentioned above was supported by a study investigating an online support group for individuals who survived the suicide of a loved one (Hollander, 2001). An analysis of the interactions revealed that many of the participants had never disclosed the secrets of their tormented minds to their social environment prior to joining the group. The emotional climate that developed in the group and the empathic understanding they received from the members provided an emotionally secure space in which they could express the feelings and thoughts that had preoccupied them since the catastrophe. Besides the emotional relief and the feeling of affiliation, the online support group assisted them in restructuring their identity, which was seriously undermined following the event. The value of the support group is exemplified in the following text written by one of the members:

> "When my son committed suicide, I experienced the same things that all other suicide families experience – friends avoiding us, people judging us [...] The grief sites on the Internet are open 24/7 so you can dump what you need to dump when you need to dump it [...]Practically everyone who visits these sites has been through it, and has some idea how bad we feel (unlike the rest of this culture) [...] I don't think I could have survived my son's suicide without the web." (Hollander, 2001, pp. 140-141)

Psychological Maintenance and the Prevention of Recurrent Hospitalization

One of the major problems involved in treating individuals suffering from chronic mental disorders is the recurrence of attacks after the termination of the treatment. This problem is typical of diseases such as schizophrenia, depression, and eating disorders in which individuals are hospitalized when the level of the symptoms rises. The treatment ends when the individual has regained his/her psychological equilibrium and can return to his/her normal routine. Unfortunately, in many cases the attacks recur, necessitating an additional period of hospitalization. This process provokes great distress and impairs the individual's chances of recovery or of improvement. In many cases, the recurrence of attacks results from a lack of either regular preventive treatment or of a supportive environment in the community.

Owing to their availability 24/7, their almost limitless accessibility, and the emotional safety afforded by the online environment, online support groups can be a valuable source of ongoing support for individuals who have been released from psychiatric hospitals. Mental health professionals have discovered the potential of online support groups to prevent re-hospitalization and consequently have begun to integrate them into their work. One example is an online support group whose aim is to prevent the re-hospitalization of adolescents and young women who suffer from eating disorders (Gulec, Moessner, Mezei, Kohls, Tury & Bauer, 2011). Another example is an online support group for individuals who were released from hospitals after receiving treatment for depression. The evaluation study showed a significantly lower number of re-hospitalizations of individuals in the group than in a control group (Bauer, Wolf, Haug & Kordy, 2011).

Suicide Prevention

Individuals who experience suicide crisis usually suffer from acute mental pain, which is manifested in a mixture of negative feelings such as grief, emptiness, disappointment, helplessness, and hopelessness. In spite of the natural urge to escape the pain, many suicidal individuals avoid seeking psychological help (Joiner, 2005), and about half of those who completed suicide were not undergoing professional treatment at the time of death (Clark & Fawcett, 1992; Isometsa, Aro, Henriksson, Heikkinen & Lonnquist, 1994). One of the explanations suggested for this irrational behavior posits that suicidal individuals are engaged in interpersonal processes eliciting loops of negative feedback that intensify the severity of their crisis (Joiner, 1995; Joiner et al., 2002). Stellrecht, Joiner, and Rudd (2006) point out that by seeking verification for their self-view, suicidal individuals engender frustration and irritation among others in their environment. This process, which augments their sense of being a burden, generates the conviction that nobody can understand or help them – and this, in turn, leads to a negative attitude toward seeking professional help.

Theoretically, this vicious circle can be broken by a supportive social environment that reacts to the ongoing suicidal messages with tolerance and understanding, and validates the mental pain. The online support group can create such an environment. The participants' own experiences with suicide crisis enable them to display genuine understanding of another person's anguish; anonymity can prevent the sense of burdensomeness that emerges in a familiar environment; and the disinhibition of self-disclosure enhances the expression of the suicidal member's deepest feelings and thoughts.

Studies examining help-seeking among suicidal individuals show that the online support group constitutes an attractive agent of assistance. One study examined the prevalence of appeals for assistance to three channels offered by the same mental health center – a volunteer-based emotional first-aid center. The results showed that 15% of the individuals who sought help from the online support group were suicidal as compared to less than 2% of those who sought assistance from the personal chat or telephone help-line (Gilat & Shahar, 2007).

Studies examining the processes occurring in the online support group shed light on the value of this environment for suicidal individuals (Gilat, 2008; Miller & Gergen, 1998): The group members give the help-seekers emotional support and avoid critical and judgmental responses almost totally. Moreover, the assistance offered to the help-seekers is not limited to emotional support, but is also evidenced by inducing cognitive change and suggesting practical ideas to cope with the distress. The advantage of the group over individual interactions in offering cognitive assistance results from the variety of perspectives to which the help-seekers are exposed. Another advantage of the group over individual assistance is the flexibility that is evident in the process (Gilat, 2008). In one case, for instance, the initial efforts of a group member to change the attitude of a suicidal member were unsuccessful, but the member adhered to her strategy – regardless of the poor results. Only the intervention of another member altered the process completely, leading to more cooperative behavior on the part of the suicidal help-seeker.

The Unique Value of Trained Volunteers

The support group operated by ERAN differs from self-aid groups in that the group is moderated by external members, namely, a team of volunteers. The moderators fulfill two functions: (1) They manage the structure and process of the group; and (2) They provide support for the group participants. Thus, the latter may receive help from both moderators and group members. This situation of dual responses to the same messages sent by troubled individuals has created a rare methodological opportunity to compare the nature of the responses sent by trained volunteers with those sent by lay members of the group. The comparison was conducted by means of two studies on the support group operated by ERAN. The aim of the first study (Gilat, Tobin & Shahar, 2011) was to identify strategies employed by the responders (either lay members or trained volunteers) in response to the messages sent to the forum by suicidal individuals. A qualitative analysis of the messages that were sent as responses yielded eight strategies employed by the responders. The strategies can be divided into three categories: *emotion-focused*, *cognitive-focused*, and *behavior-focused.*

The *emotion-focused* category comprised two strategies:

(1) A *supportive strategy*, which sought to create a personal emotional bond with the distressed individual, for example:

"I'm covering you with hugs from my heart."
"I feel your emotional turmoil."
"I pray to God to send you strength."

(2) *Offering group support,* in which the distressed individuals were invited to join the group and use it as source of support, for example:

"I invite you to join us. We are here to support, encourage, and help."

The *cognitive-focused* category comprised four strategies:

(1) *Empowerment*, which aimed to change the self-perception of the suicidal individual by raising his/her awareness of his/her internal resources, for example:

"...Your words are so vivid."
"...You have overcome the diabolical power of anorexia."

"Look at what you write to others; you know how to think positively."

(2) *Cognitive change inducement*, which focused on broadening the suicidal individual's perspective by offering an alternative meaning, reducing the perceived threat, or increasing the salience of the positive aspects of the situation, for example:

"My dear, right now you feel all alone, but this situation will not last forever; the problem is temporary and reversible."

(3) *Interpretation*, which aimed to offer a psychological explanation of the source of the problem, or to raise the user's awareness of his/her maladaptive ways of coping with the crisis, for example:

"You chose the easy solution to cope with your problems."

(4) *Persuasion*, which focused on an attempt to change the attitude of the suicidal individual by presenting logical and rational arguments against suicide, for example:

"Such a decision is irreversible",

or by presenting general beliefs about the value of life, for example:

"Life is too precious to be wasted."

The *"behavior-focused"* category comprised two strategies:

(1) *Advising*, which offered the suicidal individual practical ways of coping with the crisis, for example:

"...Try to send supportive responses to other members and you'll see that it will do you good".

(2) *Referring*, whereby the responder recommended that the suicidal individual seek professional help in addition to the support offered by the group.

The aim of the second study was to determine whether trained volunteers and lay members differ with regard to the strategies they employ in response to suicidal messages. The results demonstrated that trained volunteers utilized the following strategies significantly more frequently than lay individuals: *emotional support* (92% vs. 70%); *empowerment* (21% vs. 8%); *interpretation* (25% vs. 4%); *cognitive-change inducement* (52% vs. 10%). The only strategy that lay individuals employed more frequently than trained volunteers was *self-disclosure* (24% vs. 4%). There were no differences between the two groups as regards *persuasion*, *advising*, *referring*, and *offering group support*.

Although the present study did not evaluate the effectiveness of the interactions in terms of outcomes, from the type of strategies employed, namely, *providing emotional support*, *offering group support*, *empowering*, *suggesting a more optimistic outlook*, and *offering practical ideas* for coping with the crisis, we can assume that almost all of them are potentially helpful. The strategies mentioned above were employed more frequently by the volunteers than by the lay individuals.

In contrast, the strategy of *self-disclosure*, which was more prevalent among the lay individuals, was employed infrequently by the volunteers. Self-disclosure means that the help-givers share their personal experiences with the help-seekers. Because it conveys authenticity and genuine empathy, self-disclosure may be helpful in the framework of an online support group. On the other hand, it is fraught with danger since it has the potential to trigger suicidal ideations. This study shows that regardless of the consequences of utilizing the strategy of self-disclosure, the trained volunteers eschewed the use of this response; in so doing, they positioned themselves nearer to professionals.

The findings of this study reveal that trained volunteers differ from lay individuals when rendering emotional first aid. This is evidenced by the volunteers' use of a greater variety of assisting strategies – growth-inducing responses in particular. As a consequence of this finding, we have a more comprehensive understanding of the volunteers' unique role in crisis intervention. The rationale underlying the use of volunteers, as formulated by the pioneers of crisis intervention, foregrounds their non-professional nature, thereby enabling them to bypass the professional barriers and offer the client immediate warmth and personal involvement (McGee & Jennings, 2002).

The present study furnishes another aspect of the unique value of trained volunteers. While volunteers do indeed imbue their encounters with individuals in crisis with warmth, authenticity, and spontaneity, these are not the only attributes that they offer the help-seekers. In addition to the appropriate emotional first-aid skills they acquired during their training, volunteers have the ability to apply a therapeutic approach. Although this does not signify that they can replace professionals, they can certainly play a complementary role. This is manifested in their helpfulness in reducing the risk in critical situations or in inducing the conditions that encourage individuals in crisis to seek professional help.

The Limitations and Risks of Online Support Groups

Flaming: Internet communication is characterized by a decreased level of inhibitions vis-à-vis the direct expressions of emotions. The advantage of this feature for enhancing self-disclosure and creating a supportive atmosphere notwithstanding, it is potentially liable to sabotage the group climate via the expression of negative feelings, aggression, criticism, and judgment. By threatening the norms of a supportive atmosphere, which constitutes the basis of support groups, hostile messages can be particularly destructive in the support group environment (Alonzo & Aiken, 2004). Another source of threat is the "invasion" of strangers known as "trolls" who deliberately attempt to sabotage the group. They send aggressive and provocative messages in an attempt to shift the focus of the discussions to irrelevant subjects.

Studies examining interactions in online support groups show that flaming is rare (Gilat, 2008; Miller & Gergen, 1998). These findings suggest that that an internal control mechanism develops spontaneously in online groups and helps maintain a positive atmosphere.

Increase in negative symptoms: Many online support group participants suffer from mental disorders such as depression, anxiety, and eating disorders. By reading the messages in the group, they are exposed to contents that mirror their own mental disorders. For instance, individuals who suffer from depression read descriptions of the suffering of other members with depression. Critics of online support groups claim that the encounter with the depression of others may intensify their own experience and exacerbate their situation. This claim was corroborated in a renowned study (Coyne, 1976) in which individuals who had never suffered from depression spoke with depressive individuals and subsequently experienced a deterioration in their mood and an increase in feelings of anger and hostility. The danger of the contagious effect of online support groups has received attention in the domain of suicide crisis (Cialdini, 2003) and is explained by suicidal individuals' internal conflict between the urge to escape the mental pain on the one hand and the urge to live on the other. Messages that legitimize suicide as a solution to pain can serve to justify the suicide solution.

How do online support groups cope with this risk? The effect of disclosing negative experiences depends not only on the content of the messages, but also on the responses of the members and the moderator. If, for instance, a message expressing depression, emptiness, hopelessness, and severe self-criticism remains unanswered, it may exert a negative effect on the moods of other members who identify with it. However, if the response to such a message consists of emotional support, encouragement, and suggestions for coping with the problem, it may have a positive effect on the members.

Avoidance of seeking professional help: Some critics of self-aid groups and support groups moderated by non-professional volunteers claim that participation in the group serves as an excuse to avoid seeking professional help on the part of those who suffer from acute disorders. A meaningful and long-term improvement in such disorders (e.g., depression, anxieties, suicidal thoughts, eating disorders) necessitates knowledge and skills that are solely the purview of mental health professionals. Many individuals may avoid seeking professional help because of both the psychological price (such as shame and dependence) and the practical price associated with this type of help. Online support groups may be very attractive for these individuals because they almost entirely eliminate the price of seeking emotional assistance on the one hand, and provide immediate relief to the sufferer on the other. Such individuals may therefore use the group as a substitute for professional help and miss the opportunity to benefit from such help. It is unlikely that a valid study examining the claim that participation in online support groups comes at the expense of seeking professional therapy will be conducted. However, the experience garnered in the online support group operated by ERAN suggests that the relationship between seeking online support and seeking professional therapy is not simple. Some members reported receiving treatment in addition to their participation in the group. In most cases, the therapists encouraged them to use the online support group as an additional source of assistance. Other members commenced professional therapy, but decided to terminate it because it did not live up to their expectations. Still other members had never seen a therapist and asserted that they would not do so in the future, either. To sum up, it is reasonable to assume that some of the members would have benefited from therapy had they not been dependent on the online group; however, by and large, the link between online support groups and professional therapy is based more on completion than on competition.

"I'm Losing Control of Myself": Analysis of an Entire Thread

The value of the online support group as a source of assistance in acute situations is illustrated in the present section via an analysis of an entire interaction ("thread") that was retrieved from the online support group operated by ERAN. This is a publicly-accessible forum, moderated by trained volunteers, whose objective is to offer emotional support to anyone who needs it. Many participants are recurrent, that is, they use the forum on a regular basis and are familiar with one another, while others are one-time or infrequent visitors. The thread presented in this section developed as a result of a post sent to the forum by one of the recurrent members. The participants in the thread are the help-seeker (HS) who sent the opening message, the volunteers (V) who responded to the message, and the lay participants (LP) who also responded to the message.

> Original message: "I'm losing control of myself"
> HS: I can't control the urge to injure myself.

The help-seeker sends a very brief and focused message, devoid of any context. She does not say anything about herself, nor does she mention the reasons for her self-destructive drive. She limits the message to the immediate, dangerous situation. The succinct nature of the message can be explained by the fact that the help-seeker is well-known to many of the regular group members, who are familiar with the general context of the dramatic message. Although the help-seeker does not specify her expectations they can be deduced from the nature of the support group.

> **Volunteer A:** I know that you have the desire to harm yourself. This step may seem to you to be a solution to the pain that is engulfing you, but you know that doing yourself harm will not bring you any relief.

Two strategies can be identified in the volunteer's response. She began with an empathic message and continued with a cognitive strategy whose aim was to persuade the help-seeker to renounce her plan.

HS: I can't… It's too difficult... It's stronger than me…

The volunteer's response did not result in any change, not even a slight one; the help-seeker still adhered to her urge to harm herself. Her discourse implies that she was experiencing her destructive drive as a separate entity operating independently within her life space.

> **Volunteer A:** My dear, you're writing here – it means that you can. You have already made your move. In spite of your dominant urge, you came here first. It brings out your other voice, asking to be heard. Tell yourself: I can stop it. In small steps, little by little …"

The volunteer did not renounce her efforts in spite of the help-seeker's uncooperative response. Her second response was also cognitive-oriented, suggesting that the troubled help-seeker had an alternative outlook on her mental state. She exhorted the help-seeker to interpret the very act of appealing for assistance as an indication of control and the will to live. She also offered her practical guidelines for coping with the distress, namely, auto-suggestion (*"Tell yourself: I can stop it.")*.

> **HS:** Not anymore…

The help-seeker sent a brief but firm response, indicating that she was not in the least moved by the volunteer's messages. The response practically eliminated the likelihood of anyone offering her effective assistance.

> **LP A:** My dear, I well understand the pain and the urge and your internal debates for and against self-harm. I wish I could tell you that I succeeded in overcoming it and tell you the secret […] I can only pray for you that you'll feel better […] supporting and understanding you – J.

During this phase of the process, one of the members joined the interaction by sending a message containing nothing but understanding and support, based on her own experience with the urge to inflict self-harm. Alongside the empathy and the emotional support, a less encouraging message can be detected in this text. The fact that the responder had not succeeded in coping with the urge was liable to increase the help-seeker's anxiety.

> **HS:** This habit is terrible… I don't know how to get rid of it… I don't feel the sharp pain… my soul hurts more than the knife… I'm so scared…

While this response was not proof that the help-seeker was changing her mind regarding self-harm, the nature of her response was different than the previous responses: instead of a very succinct description of her mental state, she provided a more detailed description of her anguish. This change could enhance the process of support because it was more engaging than the brief responses; it enabled other participants to make contact with the help-seeker's internal world.

> **LP B:** I've read the thread and I'm also one of those who harm themselves. But now I've kicked the habit. I haven't done it for two years. What's the secret??? Dear, the secret is people. To talk, to get help, to vent as much as you can. Words are powerful. I know it from my own experience.

By joining the group interaction, lay member B created a sub-group of "self-harmers" operating within the global space of the support group. The message she sent was potentially valuable because she was not simply disclosing her experience with self-harm, but rather describing how she had coped with the problem successfully. Moreover, she shared the secret of her success: *"to talk, to get help, to vent as much as you can."* This "secret" reflects professional knowledge that is based on research and clinical experience. However, the lay member did not acquire this knowledge by reading professional material, but rather from her own experience. In consequence, it imbued her message with a powerful validity. Had one of the moderators written the same words, it would not have exerted such a powerful effect on the help-seeker and probably not on other members, either.

> **HS:** Other than this forum, I don't have anyone to talk to… I don't have sisters…I don't have a mother… I can't pour my heart out, so I hurt myself… I want to kick the habit, but I can't.

This message reflected an additional change in the nature of the help-seeker's reaction. For the first time since this thread began, she did not limit herself to mentioning the urge to hurt herself, but expanded on the "self" she presented to the group. She described briefly, but poignantly, a situation of acute loneliness that led to the destructive behavior. Moreover, for the first time, she expressed her wish to be cured.

> **LP B:** My dear, why don't you seek help? Everyone needs help in hard times. There are several possibilities. Love, P.
>
> **Volunteer B:** Do you see how much love you receive from the members? It doesn't solve the problem, but it tells you that you aren't alone.

The volunteer summed up a process that took place within a sub-group of "self-harmers". He/She did not mention anything about the content of the discussion, but rather reflected the process as an instrument for empowering the troubled help-seeker.

> **HS:** I thank you for your concern and for your caring. It does my heart good. Good to know that there people who care. But beyond this, I don't know if you can do anything... I don't know...

The help-seeker's closing message summarizes – briefly, but accurately – the advantages and the limitations of the online support group. Although this type of group does not engender enduring change in the individual's mental health, it affords emotional support and empowerment that may serve as a source of light that illuminates a dark world.

CONCLUSION

Individuals who choose to seek assistance from an online support group cannot only benefit from the advantages of thc online environment – which is shared by other online channels – but also exploit the gains inherent in the dynamics of groups. Interestingly enough, group processes that have been shown to possess therapeutic power in the face-to-face environment are not less powerful on the Internet. Online support groups are extremely prevalent on the Internet, and millions of people participate in self-aid groups that offer assistance in a wide variety of problem domains and are not moderated by an external agent. Trained volunteers may make a unique contribution to these groups by serving as moderators, creating a framework that increases the efficacy of the assistance provided by the group.

Chapter 7

HELPFULNESS OF EMOTIONAL FIRST AID VIA THE INTERNET

ABSTRACT

This chapter presents two studies that investigated the helpfulness of emotional first aid on the Internet. The first study examined the perceptions of 118 individuals who responded to a questionnaire pertaining to their level of satisfaction with an interaction with a volunteer via the personal chat. The results showed that 82% of them exhibited a high level of satisfaction with the chat. In addition, emotion-focused assistance was perceived to be better than cognitive and behavioral types of assistance. The second study was based on the qualitative analysis of transcripts of chats that were defined as helpful according to predetermined criteria. The analysis revealed that helpful interactions are characterized by the following components: the establishment of an emotional bond followed by the introduction of change-inducing strategies using gentle, unpretentious, non-threatening language, and adhering to an organized conversational structure.

INTRODUCTION

Evaluating the effectiveness of psychotherapy is a major issue in the field of mental health. A great deal of effort has been invested in examining the success of the various methods employed by therapists for the purposes of providing psychological assistance and identifying the factors that either enhance or inhibit a successful outcome. Evaluating the effectiveness of psychotherapy on the Internet has been particularly challenging in light of the skeptical and even opposing viewpoint regarding the very idea of offering online emotional assistance. The main argument supporting this opposing viewpoint posited that the lack of non-verbal cues precludes any possibility of attaining sufficiently high standards of client assessment and therapy (Lebow, 1998). This view challenged professionals who practiced online therapy to test the effectiveness of this type of therapy from its very onset, and to expand their endeavors in the years that followed.

Two lines of research are discernible in evaluating the effectiveness of online psychological assistance. The first focuses on the interpersonal relationships that develop between the two partners in the therapeutic encounter. The main question guiding this line of research is: Can a significant emotional bond be established between client and therapist on the Internet? Studies focusing on this question derive their inspiration from the psycho-dynamic approach, which views the formation of a "therapeutic alliance" as a precondition for successful psychotherapy (Martin, Garske & Davis, 2000). One of the earliest studies on psychotherapy on the Internet was conducted by Parks and Roberts (1998), who found that online therapy did not differ from face-to-face therapy in terms of the depth of the relationship (measured by statements such as "I feel that I can trust her in almost every aspect") and in the breadth of the relationship (measured by statements such as "From the very beginning of the meeting, we can move easily from topic to topic"). Additional studies demonstrated that the quality of the relationship between client and therapist is certainly not less meaningful, but sometimes even more so than face-to-face therapy (Cook & Doyle, 2002; Roy & Gillett, 2008).

The second line of research focuses on identifying changes in output measures of therapy conducted on the Internet such as decrease in symptoms, increase in emotional welfare, and amelioration of social functioning. Studies that were guided by this approach examined populations suffering from diverse types of distress and disorders, and furnished a great deal of evidence attesting to the success of online therapy in effecting the desired changes. For instance, participation in an online therapy group was effective in reducing the number of recurrent hospitalizations in patients who were discharged from psychiatric hospitals (Bauer, Wolf, Haug & Kordy, 2011) and in decreasing the level of symptoms in patients suffering from depression (Houston, Cooper & Ford, 2002). The success of online therapy in effecting specific changes was also demonstrated in studies evaluating therapy that was based on the cognitive-behavioral approach (CBT). Tilov and colleagues (2011) performed a random-controlled experiment that revealed a significant decrease in symptoms of depression and anxiety among patients who were receiving CBT.

Most of the studies examining the effectiveness of online assistance were conducted in the context of professional therapy. Empirical evidence on the effectiveness of the emotional first aid provided online by trained volunteers is scarce. The present chapter evaluates the helpfulness of personal chats as a source of emotional first aid provided by trained volunteers. This evaluation was conducted by means of two separate examinations that were based on methodologies.

The first examination focused on the help-seekers' perspective as regards the effect of the chat on their well-being. For the purpose of gathering the data, the help-seekers completed a structured post-chat questionnaire.

The second examination focused on the evaluation of expert professional judges as regards the benefit of the chat to the help-seekers. The judges analyzed transcripts of chats that fulfilled the criteria of helpfulness such as the direct report of the help-seeker toward the end of the chat or changes in the help-seeker's perception during the course of the chat. While this methodology does not provide direct evidence of the effectiveness of the chat, it can shed light on the processes that increase the likelihood of helpful outcomes of online interactions between troubled individuals and trained volunteers.

Three research questions were posed: (1) How do online help-seekers perceive the helpfulness of interactions with the volunteers via the personal chat? (2) What are the reasons for selecting the personal chat as a source of assistance? (3) What are the characteristics of helpful interactions in the personal chat?

The first two questions were examined using a quantitative questionnaire, while the third question was examined by means of a qualitative analysis of the transcripts. The study was conducted in the context of ERAN (the Israeli Association for Emotional First Aid), a mental health service offering emotional assistance via telephone and the Internet. The assistance is provided by volunteers who receive training and supervision from professionals (see Chapter 1). The methodology employed to evaluate the impact of the personal chats on the help-seekers was a client satisfaction survey. This methodology is based on the subjective reports of the clients, and does not enable conclusions to be drawn regarding the question of whether any objective changes occurred following the chats. Thus, the study measured the "perceived helpfulness" of the chat rather than its effectiveness.

Helpfulness of Emotional First Aid on the Internet: The Clients' Perspective

Method

Data: The sample consisted of 118 help-seekers who contacted the personal chat – 79 females (67%) and 39 males (33%). *Age:* 12-56 with a mean of 22.73 and standard deviation of 7.77. *Occupation:* school pupils – 36%, soldiers – 7%, students – 18%, adults (employed) – 23%, adults (not employed) – 16%. *Previous contact with ERAN:* The participants were asked if they had sought online assistance from ERAN in the past via any of the three channels – personal chat, email, or support group. The results showed that 73% had sought assistance via the personal chat, 31% via email, and 22% via the online support group. (The percentages do not add up to 100 because help-seekers sometimes apply for more than one channel of assistance). *Professional treatment:* Over half of the online help-seekers (54%) reported a history of psychological treatment, and 30% reported a history of psychiatric treatment.

Instrument: Data were gathered by means of a questionnaire that was designed for the purpose of the study and included the following sections: (1) personal characteristics of the help-seekers; (2) satisfaction with the chat, including general satisfaction (*"I am satisfied with the personal chat"*); emotional impact of the chat (*"The chat helped me feel better"*); cognitive impact (*"The chat helped me understand my situation more clearly"*); behavioral impact (*"I will implement the advice offered by the volunteer"*); impact on self-disclosure (*"I told the volunteers things about myself that I had not told [anyone] before"*); and (3) two open questions: (a) "How did the chat with the volunteer affect you?" (b) "Why did you choose the chat as a channel of seeking assistance?" In order to validate the questionnaire, three expert judges (mental health professionals with experience in online assistance) were requested to read the questionnaire and comment on the content of the items, namely, their relevance to evaluating helpfulness, and on the language, namely, the clarity of the items and their comprehensibility.

Procedure: Data were collected over a four-month period in 2012. At the end of each chat, ERAN's volunteers asked the help-seekers whether they were willing to participate in a study whose objective was to evaluate their satisfaction with the chat. The volunteers explained that the help-seeker's role was to complete an online questionnaire by entering a link and submitting a response. It was stressed that the response was anonymous, the data would be used for research purposes only, and participation in the study was voluntary. During the four-month period, 1,200 chats occurred (after the exclusion of recurrent help-seekers who were included only once). In 300 cases (e.g., suicidal help-seekers), the volunteers did not ask the help-seekers to complete the questionnaire. The number of questionnaires that were completed was 118, constituting 13% of the 900 help-seekers who were requested to do so.

RESULTS

Reasons to Select the Personal Chat

In order to examine the reasons for selecting the personal chat as an environment for seeking emotional assistance, the participants were requested to respond to an open question: "Why did you contact ERAN via the personal chat?" A content analysis of the responses was performed by two psychologists who are experienced in online assistance. The analysis yielded nine categories of reasons to use the chat. Table 1 presents the categories and their frequencies. The frequencies do not add up to 100 because thc categories were not mutually exclusive, that is, more than one reason could be identified in a single response.

Table 1. Reasons for selecting the personal chat (N=94)

Category	Frequency (%)
Elimination of emotional barriers	35
Anonymity and confidentiality	28
Preference for written communication	18
Quality of volunteers	16
Availability and immediacy of receiving assistance	14
Additional advantages of the medium	12

a. *Elimination of emotional barriers:* The environment in which the chat occurs lowers the emotional barriers and enhances openness and self-disclosure.

"When I talk in the chat, I am willing to say things that I do not say in verbal speech, so when I talk in the chat I am more open."

"The fear of people fades away beyond the words that are typed on the keyboard."

"In the chat, I am not nervous and not shy, so I can describe my case in the best way."

b. *Anonymity and confidentiality:* The option to remain anonymous with one's chat partner affords the emotional security necessary for the disclosure of personal distress.

"The fact that I can remain anonymous and talk in a place where I am not judged helps me cope with myself better."

"I chose the chat because everything is anonymous and you can talk about anything, even more than with your best friend."

"I don't feel safe to talk about it with my family or friends, and the telephone is too direct and they can understand exactly who I am. In the chat, everything is discreet, so I feel safer with the volunteer."

c. *Preference for written communication:* Two advantages of writing emerged from the participants' responses. One of them stressed the emotional aspect, stating that writing provides an appropriate emotional climate for expressing emotions – more than talking does. The second advantage stresses the cognitive contribution of writing to the advancement and enrichment of thinking.

"I am very good at writing! Very weak at talking. It's difficult for me to express my emotions by talking, and I do it very well by writing!"

"What I like about the chat is the writing. It helps me to think with the volunteer while I'm writing and to get to the insights."

d. *Quality of the volunteers:* Selecting the chat is explained by the quality of ERAN's volunteers, which is perceived as high from both professional and human perspectives.

"I only call ERAN regularly because I know that I'll be in good hands."

"When the volunteers I know respond to me and help me find the exact words to describe what I feel, it makes me happier than anything in the world. The letters that build the words are the same, but the words of each volunteer are unique and give me the opportunity to encounter different points of view from the best people in Israeli society."

"In my view, you're angels. The answers are so helpful and come from a good and genuine place. Most important is the understanding and the thinking that give correct directions."

e. *Availability and immediacy of receiving assistance:* Eliminating the barriers of time and distance enables the help-seekers to receive emotional assistance anytime, anywhere.

"I felt an urgent need to talk about something that I can't talk about with any of my friends."

"I was too shy to tell my story, but I needed to consult someone because it was very urgent."

"I decided to use the chat because I'm now studying in the United States and I can't use the hotline."

f. *Additional advantages of the medium:* This category includes additional advantages of the personal chat, particularly the ability to control the pace of the communication and the ability to engage in other activities while chatting.

"It's convenient from the point of view of thc pace."

"I sought help regarding a friend who threatened to kill herself. I could talk to you and to the friend at the same time."

"I can listen to music while I'm chatting."

Satisfaction with the Chat

The help-seekers were requested to rate their level of satisfaction with various aspects of the personal chat. Table 2 presents the means, standard deviations, and frequency distributions (in %) for each statement of the questionnaire. The statements are presented in a descending order of satisfaction.

The results reveal that the level of the help-seekers' general satisfaction with the personal chat was high. More than 80% of them were satisfied with the online interaction with the volunteer and reported a high degree of willingness to continue seeking assistance from the chat if the need arose. A closer observation of the results reveals that although the satisfaction with specific aspects of the chat was lower than the general satisfaction, it was still quite high. For instance, 60–70% of the respondents were satisfied with the helpfulness of the chat as regards the emotional aspect, 50–60% reported a high level of satisfaction with the cognitive contribution of the chat, and 40–50%were satisfied with the practical contribution of the chat. In addition, 70–90% of the respondents were satisfied with the conduct of the volunteer.

Table 2. Descriptive statistics of help-seekers' satisfaction with the personal chat

Statement	% of agreement			Mean	SD
	Low	Medium	High		
The volunteer did not judge or criticize me	6.8	3.4	89.6	4.53	0.97
The language of the volunteer was appropriate	4.3	3.5	92.2	4.49	0.89
I will turn to ERAN again if I need assistance	5.1	10.3	84.6	4.46	0.98
The volunteer was clear and understandable	5.2	5.2	89.5	4.43	0.93
Generally, I am satisfied with the chat	7.7	10.3	82.0	4.21	1.07
I told the volunteers things that I do not tell anybody	11.3	13.0	75.7	4.18	1.16
I felt understood by the volunteer	9.5	13.0	77.4	4.08	1.10
I am satisfied with the pace of the chat	12.9	16.4	70.7	4.03	1.16
I am satisfied with the duration of the chat	13.0	16.5	70.5	4.02	1.20
The chat helped me feel better	12.8	17.1	70.1	3.93	1.18
The chat helped me feel that I am not alone	20.7	10.3	68.9	3.84	1.35
The chat helped me feel stronger	15.4	19.7	65.0	3.73	1.20
The chat helped me see my situation more clearly	19.3	24.6	56.1	3.55	1.30
The chat provided me with useful information	20.5	26.5	53.0	3.51	1.22
I received practical ideas for coping with my problem	26.5	23.1	50.4	3.45	1.37
The chat gave me a different perspective on my situation	26.5	26.5	47.0	3.33	1.28
I will implement the advice that was given to me	27.4	25.6	47.0	3.38	1.35
The chat helped me view my situation differently	26.5	26.5	47.0	3.33	1.28
The chat will help me solve the problem	32.5	25.4	42.1	3.09	1.35

Four general categories of perceived helpfulness were derived from the specific items in the questionnaire. The reliability of the categories was tested by Cronbach's alpha. Table 3 presents the categories and the values of reliability.

Table 3. Categories of perceived helpfulness

Category	Items	Alpha
Emotional change	• The chat helped me feel better	0.85
	• The chat helped me feel that I am not alone	
	• The chat helped me feel stronger	
Cognitive change	• The chat helped me see my situation more clearly	0.86
	• The chat provided me with useful information	
	• The chat gave me a different perspective on my situation	
	• I received practical ideas for coping with my problem	0.89
Behavioral change	• I will implement the advice that was given to me	
	• The chat will help me solve the problem	
Enhancing openness	• I told the volunteers things that I do not tell anybody	(one item)

Four measures of the perceived impact of the chat were constructed by averaging the responses to the statements included in each category (except for "enhancing openness", which consisted of a single item). A higher score in the measure indicates a higher degree of change. To determine whether there were differences between the domains of change, a uni-variate ANOVA with repeated measures was conducted with the domain of change as the independent variable and the degree of change as the dependent variable. The analysis yielded a significant effect of the domain ($F(3,112) = 25.11$, $p < .001$). Post-hoc multiple comparisons ($P < .05$) revealed significant differences among the four domains, so that the increase in openness was significantly higher than the emotional change, which was significantly higher than the cognitive change, which was significantly than the behavioral change. The perceived changes in the four domains are presented in Figure 1.

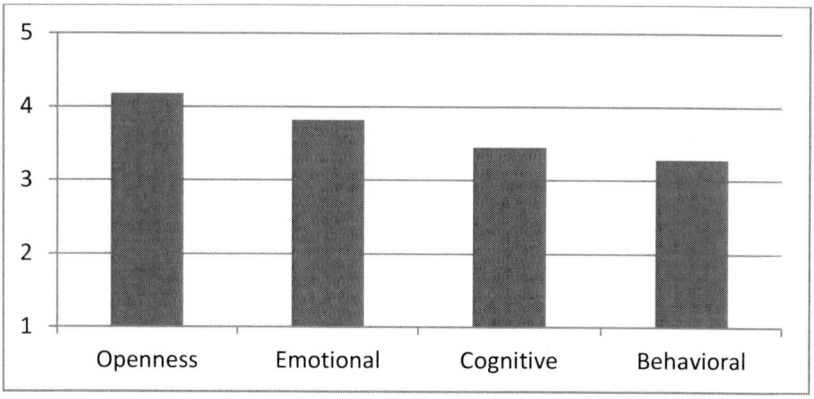

Figure 1. Changes in the four domains following the personal chat.

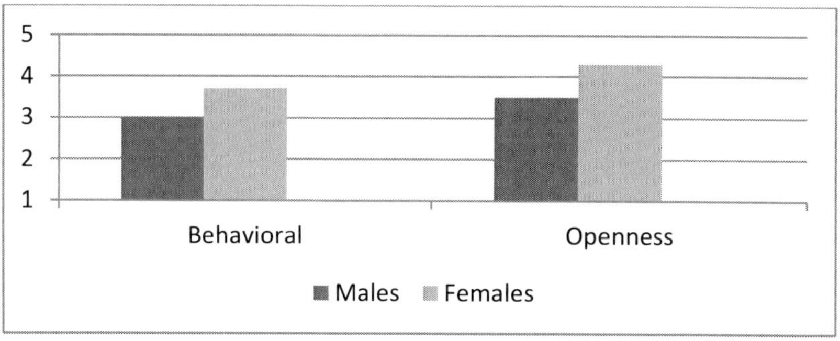

Figure 2. Significant changes in two domains among male and female help-seekers.

Analyses of variance were performed in order to examine the relationship between the perceived change and the help-seekers' personal characteristics. Only the help-seeker's gender was significantly related to the perceived change, while the other characteristics (occupation, previous contact/s with ERAN, and professional treatment) were not. As regards gender, a multi-variate analysis revealed significant differences between males and females with respect to the impact of the chat on behavioral change ($F(1,113) = 2.03$, $p <.05$) and on enhancing openness ($F(1,113) = 1.93$, $p <.05$). Figure 2 presents the means of the perceived change in these domains by gender of the help-seeker. The figure shows that with respect to the behavioral aspect and to openness, female help-seekers perceived the degree of change as higher than male help-seekers.

The Impact of the Chat on the Help-seeker: Analysis of Responses to Open-ended Questions

In order to examine the impact of the chat on the help-seekers in greater depth, the respondents were asked to answer two open-ended questions: (1) "How did the chat affect you?" (2) "What actions will you take following the chat?" A content analysis of the responses was conducted by two psychologists experienced in online counseling.

The Effect of the Chat

The analysis yielded seven types of positive effect (enhancing effects) and three types of negative effect or limitation of the chat (inhibiting effects). Table 4 presents the labels of the categories and their frequencies in percentages. The percentages do not add up to 100 because more than one category may be evident in a single response.

Table 4. Enhancing and inhibiting effects of the personal chat (N=119)

Enhancing effects	Frequency (%)
Emotional and social support	49
Reinforcing a chosen strategy of action	14
Cognitive change	13
Behavioral change	8
Multi-dimensional effect	6
Inhibiting effects	
Dissatisfaction with the volunteer's attention	2
Judgmental attitude of the volunteer	1
Lack of solution to the problem	1

Enhancing Effects

Emotional and social support: The core of the emotional support, as reflected by the responses, is the help-seeker's feeling that he/she is not alone. The volunteers succeeded in invoking this feeling by accepting the help-seeker's experience non-judgmentally. They were attentive to the help-seekers, encouraged them to share their feelings and thoughts, and validated their feelings:

> "The feeling that the volunteer understood me helped me very much [...] I felt that I am not alone and I told him things that I've never told [anyone] before."
>
> "I realized that someone understands me and wants to help me, coming from a non-judgmental point of view."
>
> "The volunteer understood me. She did not object to what I said, did not judge me, she was simply there for me."

Reinforcing a chosen strategy of action: This type of assistance was evident in the reinforcement of an idea or a line of action that the help-seeker had thought about:

> "The chat helped me gain reassurance regarding my situation, feel better with myself. I feel threatened by a friend who is probably angry with me and I'm trying to avoid a conflict. I gained reassurance that the friend's anger is not justified and his efforts to take control of my life are not legitimate."
>
> "They told me things that I know, but if you hear it from somebody else, it sounds different."

Cognitive change: The enhancing effect of the chat manifested itself in creating a change in the help-seeker's self-perception or providing an alternative, optimistic interpretation to the problem he/she raised:

> "After the chat, I think differently about the situation. It helped me understand that I'm not alone and that I'm strong."
>
> "The thing that helped me in the chat was that when I was talking about the bad things in my life, the volunteer made me talk about the good things, my hobbies and the good reasons to be happy."
>
> "The chat organized things in my head and gave me points to think about."

Behavioral change: The chat furnished the help-seekers with the necessary tools such as advice, information, and ideas for coping and for effecting a practical change:

> "The chat really helped me. It showed me how to get away from my situation."
>
> "She gave me a practical solution, told me where to call."
>
> "The chat made me help myself overcome my difficulty. The volunteer gave me tools."

Multi-dimensional effect: The positive effect of the chat was evident in several types of assistance:

> "What helped me is the knowledge that there is someone who really cares about me, who asks because he really wants to know the answer, who shows me the way but does not walk instead of me, someone who really understands my difficulty, who reveals his own feelings and validates mine, someone who says good and constructive words and also puts me in my place when I'm wrong."

Inhibiting Effects

Dissatisfaction with the volunteer's attention: Some help-seekers felt that they did not receive the volunteer's full attention:

> "I felt that in spite of the volunteer's good intentions, he was not completely with me and was probably busy chatting with other users."
>
> "I felt that the volunteer wanted to end the chat because she had other people waiting for her."

Judgmental attitude of the volunteer:

> "The volunteer was very judgmental and not sensitive to my experience."

No solution to the problem:

> "I was disappointed because I did not get [any] practical ideas that could help me."

Taking Post-chat Actions

Another perspective of the helpfulness of the chat is the clients' decision to take actions that can potentially improve their well-being. It is logical to assume that a single chat cannot bring about long-term changes in the help-seeker's condition. However, a single conversation with the volunteer can create the conditions for taking actions that will eventually lead to longer-term changes. In their training, the volunteers are instructed to encourage the help-seekers to take actions such as undergoing professional therapy. In order to examine this aspect of helpfulness, the clients were requested to describe the actions they intended to take. A content analysis of the 80 responses yielded four categories. Table 5 presents the labels of the categories and their frequencies in percentages. The percentages do not add up to 100 because more than one category may be evident in a single response.

Table 5. Taking post-chat actions (N=80)

Intended action	Frequency (%)
Turning to non-formal agents for support	28
Consultation with a professional	28
Implementing ideas and suggestions	39
No specific action	23

Exemplary Quotations for Each Intended Action

Turning to non-formal agents for support:

"I'll talk to people who are close to me."
"I'll tell my parents what's on my mind."

Consultation with a professional:

"I'll go to the school counselor to talk about my eating disorders."
"I'll continue the therapy that I decided to stop."

Implementing ideas and suggestions:

"I'll take the volunteer's advice and I'll remember what she said, for example, to spend time on things that make me happy and not on things that make me cry."

"One of the actions that I'll take following the chat is to continue doing comforting things (such as riding my bike), try to think calmly about the quarrel with my friend, and try to go on with my routine."

No specific action:

"I won't take specific action, but I'll return to the chat if I need to."

"I won't take any action because they didn't suggest anything, they just listened to me."

HELPFULNESS OF EMOTIONAL FIRST AID ON THE INTERNET: AN EXPERT'S PERSPECTIVE

METHOD

Data

The qualitative analysis of the helpful chats was based on eight transcripts that were selected according to several helpfulness criteria. Each of the eight chats fulfilled at least one of the following criteria:

Emotional change: The emotional indication of helpfulness is a particularly positive experience associated with the connection with the volunteer, which is manifested in the help-seeker's gratitude and a feeling of personal empowerment:

"You're great! I hope you succeed in everything you do"; "I'm sending you a blessing for the rest of your life"; "I came here and understood that there are good people in the world"; "I can say 'thank you' again, but these words are too small…I don't know how to express it, so I'll simply say that it was really meaningful for me, I appreciate what you did for me, and I wish you o-n-l-y all the best."

Cognitive change: The cognitive indication for helpfulness is a change in the help-seeker's thinking, which is manifested in the creation of a broad and realistic self-perception:

> "I realized that in order to be happy, I must face my past and be able to accept it. I have to muster my strengths, stop being afraid, and start coping."

Behavioral change: The behavioral indication for helpfulness is a reversal of plans to engage in a maladaptive type of behavior such as self-harm. One suicidal help-seeker wrote at the beginning of the chat:

> "You're probably the last man I'll talk to. I'm going in the other direction, I'm tired of everything",

and at the end of the chat,

> "You saved me, you're an angel."

Changes in physical symptoms:

> "I'm certainly more relaxed, my breathing is less heavy, I feel much better."

Data Analysis

The analysis of the transcripts was performed using a qualitative methodology in which two approaches were applied – a psychology-focused approach and a language-focused approach. The psychology-focused approach sought to identify the interpersonal processes that occurred between the help-seeker and the volunteer and increased the chances for a successful outcome of the interaction. This analysis was performed by two mental health professionals with experience in online counseling. The language-focused approach sought to identify the linguistic resources employed by both parties that could contribute to the helpfulness of the chat. This analysis was performed by two experts in discourse analysis. Neither of the two types of analysis was guided by predetermined theoretical categories of helpfulness; rather, they reflected a free search of the data with respect to themes that could be associated with the helpfulness of the chat.

Characteristics of Helpful Interactions

Strategies Aimed at Forming Relationships

Emotional support: The emotional support was evidenced by the feelings expressed by the help-seekers, namely, that they were not alone and that there was someone to help them bear their burden of agony. The emotional support was provided by reflecting the help-seeker's feelings, sending empathic messages, and creating an emotional bond with the help-seeker: *"It sounds really difficult. I'm not even saying that I understand because I assume that what you're feeling really is unbearable"; "Let's try to look at it together, OK?"*

Containing: Within the context of the personal chat, 'containing' refers to the creation of an emotional space in which the help-seeker feels safe enough to disclose inner experiences, including threatening ones such as thoughts of death, self-criticism, and the urge to harm him/herself. Containing is a powerful vehicle for creating emotional intimacy with the volunteer because it affords the help-seeker an opportunity to present him/herself as he/she is, without masks, and without the risk of suffering rejection or receiving a judgmental response. The following interaction is taken from a chat with a girl suffering from AN:

> **HS:** I want to die, I can't suffer any more, I want to cut myself so badly… It seems to me that after this chat I'll disappear.
>
> **Volunteer:** Tell me a little about what you're going through.

During this initial phase of the interaction, the volunteer encourages the help-seeker to get in touch with the dark and painful aspects of her inner world, and does not exhibit a judgmental attitude such as amazement, contradict the girl's messages, or attempt to alter her wishes. (He will try to do so later, after the emotional bond and trust are developed.)

Empowerment: The strategy of empowerment seeks to effect a change in the help-seeker's self-perception by stressing his/her strengths and showing appreciation of his/her abilities:

> "Well, first of all, I think you're very brave and strong because many girls in your situation wouldn't even admit that they have a problem. You understand it and want to help yourself, and this is a strong voice of life."
>
> "I want to tell you that because of your difficulties and your psychiatric history, all the achievements that you mentioned are enormous."

"They probably have a wonderful father from whom they inherited this ability. You're a real heroine."

Controlled self-disclosure: The volunteer's self-disclosure is evidenced in the chat by the fact that he shares his personal feelings, thoughts, and experiences with the help-seeker. The analysis revealed that the volunteer's self-disclosure enhances intimacy and helps build up trust by removing the asymmetrical status barrier and presenting the volunteer as human:

Volunteer: When I was your age, I was deep in depression, everything was black, and I didn't see any way out of it. Then I decided to see a therapist and things changed.

Volunteer: I also experienced loss – both my parents died within a period of two years. It was very painful.

HS: How did you cope with it?

Compliance with a basic need of the help-seeker: In some cases, the volunteer complies completely with the help-seeker's primary emotional needs, namely, to be hugged, to feel emotionally secure:

HS: I've got nobody, I want to die, who will care? Nobody.

Volunteer: I am here with you and although we don't know each other, I care. I am with you, my attention is only for you.

HS: Promise me that you love me and you'll send me a protective hug so that nothing hurts me.

Volunteer: I promise you that I love you and I'll send you a hug, particularly in the difficult moments that attack you sometimes.

A break in the chat: The analysis of the transcripts revealed an unconventional means employed by some volunteers in order to foster the emotional bond with the help-seeker, namely, a break during the chat, after which the two parties resumed their dialogue. Such a break afforded the help-seeker an opportunity to process the feelings and ideas that emerged during the conversation. Since the volunteer remained in the background and was available to continue the chat, the break was not experienced as abandonment, but rather as a continuation of the relationship via another mode of communication. The following example is taken from a chat with a girl who was experiencing the urge to injure herself:

Volunteer: I know that it's very difficult for you, and I want to be with you, and I suggest that we take a break and continue the chat in about 15 minutes.

HS: I'll go smoke a cigarette.

Volunteer: My heart is with you even when we are not talking.

HS (after 20 minutes): I went out for a breath of air and here I am. Don't worry, I won't do anything stupid.

In some cases, the idea of taking a break came from the help-seeker, and the volunteer cooperated with it. The following example is taken from a chat with a woman who complained of severe anxiety:

HS: Can you wait until I make myself a cup of coffee?

Volunteer: I'm here, take your time, it'll do you good, I'll wait for you.

HS (after ten minutes): I'm back. Thank you.

It should be noted that the option of taking a break during the conversation is feasible owing to the technical features of the online environment, which enables the participants to take a break without ending the chat. This option is less convenient in face-to-face or telephonic communication.

Strategies Aimed at Inducing a Change

Broadening the perspective: The analysis of the helpful chats revealed that the volunteers employed a cognitive strategy that sought to broaden the help-seeker's perspective. The purpose of this strategy was to encourage the help-seeker stress positive and optimistic aspects rather than negative and threatening ones:

Volunteer (to a student who complained about feeling depressed): *What are the good things that have happened?*

HS: *First, no one in my family is ill, no one died, and no one is dying. In addition, I had several exams which I passed OK and perhaps I'll go on a vacation when the exams are over.*

Volunteer (writing to a young woman who described herself as having two opposing faces): *Can you expand on the description of the one who is constructive and developing?*

Suicidal man: *I wanted to hang myself but I chickened out at the last minute and couldn't do it.*

Volunteer: *You didn't chicken out – on the contrary, at the last moment you overcame your pain and regained control.*

Normalization: This strategy seeks to decrease the negative meaning that the help-seeker attributes to the problem by stressing the normative nature of the situation. The focus of the problem shifts from the individual level to the social level:

Volunteer: It's true for a lot of people. They reject compliments from others and intensify criticism.

Volunteer: Is there anyone who doesn't have several parts to his personality? It's not unusual at all.

Empathic confrontation: In this strategy, the volunteer presents a stance that is explicitly opposed to that of the help-seeker in order to encourage the latter to re-evaluate his/her previous view, which the volunteer considers inadequate. The strategy of confrontation is used in a later phase of the conversation, when the volunteer feels that an alliance has been established and the help-seeker will respond in a cooperative way rather than reject the message with its overtones of confrontation:

Volunteer: You are presenting a black and white situation. Either everything is OK or nothing is OK. May I suggest a different way of looking at things?

Linguistic Characteristics

The discourse analysis revealed the language employed by the volunteers to be unpretentious and familiar –language that engenders intimacy and trust. It is gentle language, the opposite of the language that is used for giving orders, which may cause the help-seeker to shut down. The unpretentiousness of the language is evident in the use of 'moderating' and everyday expressions such as "a little", "in a way", "probably", in personal appeals such as "believe me", "please, my dear", and in the use of conditional expressions (if …then), which increase trust and invite the help-seeker to consider the volunteer's messages as suggestions rather than as instructions issued by a superior. Examples of each aspect of the language employed by the volunteers are presented below.

Unpretentious language is characterized by the use of words and expressions that convey modesty:

"Believe me...try not to think of her but think of the good parts to which you are probably connected."

"Can you please drop the 'I must'?"

"Natalie dear, I think that you can accept yourself and be proud of yourself even if your grades are good and not excellent."

"My dear, I promise you that everything can be solved."

Familiar language is characterized by the use of words and expressions that increase understanding and empathy:

"I understand how you feel."

"Yes, I'm familiar with this approach."

"I'm sorry to hear it, my dear."

"I'm familiar with this situation. I also had a friend..."

"I can hear your pain."

Conditional sentences: The use of conditional expressions and sentences moderates thc language, preventing it from being unequivocal and absolute. It is language that invites the help-seeker to choose among alternatives rather than being presented with a single, uncompromising solution:

"If you receive professional treatment, you'll be able to think more clearly and think of a solution."

"If your relationship is very good, then I think you'll tell her what happened."

"If you are excited, then it means that you are in contact with these parts, you don't reject them, they're probably part of you."

The Structure of the Conversation

In most chats, a three-part structure could be identified: the beginning of the conversation, the main part, and the conclusion of the conversation. The beginning and the conclusion were rather similar in the different chats, while the main part depended on the specific characteristics of the interaction.

The beginning of the chat is characterized by containing, empathic, and inviting messages from the volunteer, encouraging the help-seeker to continue the dialogue. Another characteristic of the beginning is the use of questions whose purpose is to increase the help-seeker's openness:

> "Yes."
> "I'm here to listen."
> "I see."
> "It must have been a difficult experience."
> "Who did you turn to?"
> "What do you mean by 'last'?"
> "Did something happen today?"
> "Can you tell me a little about your feelings?"

The main part of the chat could be characterized by two orientations: providing emotional support and employing change-inducing strategies. In all cases, the establishment of a supportive atmosphere preceded the change-inducing effort.

The conclusion of the interaction was characterized by the presentation of a positive, optimistic, and challenging horizon:

> "Look at it as a challenge, as an adventure, not as a must or a threat."
> "Try to see the thesis you have to submit as something interesting, something good."

DISCUSSION

The present chapter focuses on an evaluation of the helpfulness of interactions between online help-seekers and trained volunteers via the personal chat and the identification of the factors that enhance or inhibit the successful outcome of the interaction. This evaluation was conducted on the basis of two different perspectives: that of the help-seekers, who completed a structured questionnaire, and that of the expert judges, who interpreted transcripts that were defined as helpful.

The data revealed the help-seekers' high level of satisfaction with the chat. Over 80% of them were generally satisfied and wrote that they would select the chat as a source of assistance in the future. This high level of satisfaction is consistent with previous studies that evaluated the perceived helpfulness of online assistance in professional therapy and reported that clients evaluated the quality of therapeutic relationships as high (Cook & Doyle, 2002; Parks & Roberts, 1998). The present findings demonstrate that the helpfulness of online assistance can be expanded to the context of the emotional first aid provided by trained volunteers.

A closer examination of the help-seekers' responses revealed that the online interaction with the volunteer enhanced changes in the emotional, cognitive, and behavioral domains. The emotional change was evidenced by an improvement in the help-seeker's emotional well-being by providing him/her with a supportive environment and engendering a feeling that he/she was not alone. The cognitive change manifested itself in the adoption of an alternative view of the stressful situation that was more optimistic than the previous perspective. The behavioral change was exhibited in the acceptance of tools for making decisions or for taking specific actions. The quantitative analysis revealed that the emotional contribution was perceived as higher than the cognitive and the behavioral contributions. This finding can be explained by the fact that the emotional change results – at least partly – from the interpersonal relationship that evolved between the troubled help-seeker and the supportive volunteer, signifying that its impact can be immediate, whereas cognitive or behavioral changes require more time in order for them to be processed and implemented.

An examination of the relationship between the personal characteristics of the help-seekers and the perceived helpfulness of the chat yielded only one significant finding, namely, that the contribution of the chat to emotional well-being was perceived as higher among females than among males. This finding is consistent with previous studies, showing that females derive more benefit from professional therapy than males (Chen, Jordan & Thompson, 2006. In view of the higher frequency of females seeking online help from ERAN (see Chapter 3), it may be concluded that females not only exhibit a higher degree of willingness to seek help, but also exploit the assistance in a more effective manner.

Another perspective regarding the helpfulness of the chat was based on help-seekers' reports regarding their plans to take specific actions following the chat. The qualitative analysis revealed two kinds of actions: (1) Seeking emotional support from their informal environment and as well as from formal agents such as therapists and school counselors – a line of action that can be viewed as an indication of effectiveness in light of ERAN's defined role as a mental health service. Since ERAN offers short-term assistance, one of its objectives is to pave the way for seeking professional therapy; and (2) Following advice and implementing ideas that were suggested by the volunteer, such as methods of relaxation, pursuing voluntary activities, or renewing old contacts.

Evaluating the helpfulness of the chats from the help-seekers' perspective on the basis of the structured questionnaire furnished evidence pertaining to the outcome of the interaction between them and the volunteers. Generally, this outcome was characterized by a high level of satisfaction, and was evident specifically in changes that occurred in their emotional well-being, cognitive outlooks, or behavioral aspects. In order to bring to light the processes that created these changes, we applied an in-depth qualitative analysis to the transcripts of chats that were defined as successful. This analysis yielded four components that can explain the helpful outcome: strategies for establishing an emotional bond, strategies for effecting change, the use of linguistic resources, and adherence to a typical structure of the interaction.

Establishing an emotional bond: Almost all the chats that were analyzed revealed three strategies employed by the volunteers in the initial phase of the interaction for the purpose of establishing an emotional bond with the help-seekers: containing, lending emotional support, and empowering. Containing was evidenced by the creation of an emotional space in which the help-seeker felt secure enough to present his/her authentic self and disclose experiences that could be threatening and painful. Emotional support was delivered by the volunteer via explicit messages conveying empathic understanding. Empowerment was manifested in the identification of the help-seeker's internal resources that came to the fore in the chat, and in the help-seeker's awareness of them.

In addition to the three above-mentioned strategies, which are well-known in the context of psychotherapy, the volunteers employed two other strategies that are unique to the context of emotional first aid. The first is compliance with the primary emotional needs of the help-seeker – the need for love and emotional security. Compliance with these needs was evidenced by direct and explicit expressions of affection such as sending a hug or using words retrieved from the semantic field of close relationships (e.g., “my dear”). The use of total compliance with emotional needs is probably the result of two factors: the context of emotional first aid and the characteristics of the online environment. As regards the type of assistance, emotional first aid aims to provide support and encouragement by means of a single encounter with a troubled individual. Thus, the help-giver can be more lavish in his/her use of emotional expressions than professional therapists, who are expected to observe limits in their relationships with clients. As regards the environment, communication on the Internet is characterized by the disinhibition of emotional expressions (Suler, 2004). It is reasonable to assume that a sentence such as "I love you" would not have been uttered by a volunteer during a telephone interaction with a caller, whereas it is normative on the Internet.

The second unique strategy involves taking a short break during the conversation with the help-seeker –a break upon which both participants agree –and resuming the conversation afterwards. At first glance, such a break seems liable to interrupt the continuity and jeopardize the successful outcome of the interaction. However, the analysis of the transcripts revealed that it actually enhanced the quality of the relationship and contributed to the help-seeker's ability to feel at ease. The value of the break can be explained by the fact that the volunteer remains available, while the help-seeker, far from experiencing a sense of abandonment, takes the opportunity to calm down and process the conversation that occurred beforehand.

By employing emotion-focused strategies, the volunteers afforded the troubled help-seeker the experience of an emotional bond, of belonging. Such an experience is helpful in creating a sense of security that is endowed with therapeutic value. The process of creating an emotional bond is widely used in the field of professional therapy and is known as creating a 'therapeutic alliance'. Studies have shown that such an alliance is vital for the success of the therapy (e.g., Horvath & Luborsky, 1993). The present study shows that creating an experience of alliance is not dependent upon a continuous process and can be accomplished during a single encounter that occurs in the online environment.

Nevertheless, there is a difference between the two contexts of emotional assistance in the meaning of the term 'therapeutic alliance'. In the ongoing process that takes place in professional psychotherapy, the therapeutic alliance creates the conditions for the occurrence of stable changes in the client's emotional well-being and social adaptation. The single-session encounter that takes place in the context of emotional first aid, however, does not facilitate such changes, but is sufficient to enable the help-seeker to experience emotional security, which serves as a buffer against the hazardous effects of acute loneliness on his/her mental health.

Change-inducing strategies: The analysis of the transcripts revealed that the volunteers employed a wide variety of strategies whose objective was to effect a cognitive change by suggesting an alternative meaning for the stress-evoking situation or for the internal resources of the help-seeker. Cognitive-focused strategies, which are widely used in professional therapy, did not originate in the online environment. They constitute the core of the cognitive approach to therapy, which is one of the most commonly-applied approaches in the face-to-face environment. However, the online environment offers conditions that are more suitable for the implementation of cognitive strategies. Its major advantage is the presence of the written text during the help-giver's interaction with the client. Since the essence of the cognitive approach is attributing an alternative meaning to the client's thinking, the help-giver's ability to read the products of this thinking and make use of this text (e.g., by using quotations from it) during the encounter with the help-seeker is highly advantageous.

Linguistic characteristics: The value of language in promoting the helpfulness of the interactions that occur during the personal chat is anchored in the cardinal role that language plays in interpersonal communication. Language is particularly valuable for the study of interpersonal communication on the Internet owing to the lack of nonverbal cues (Crystal, 2000). Nonverbal cues such as facial expressions and eye contact are necessary for the interpretation of verbal messages in face-to-face communication. The communication in the online environment is compensated for the lack of these cues in several ways. One of the principal ways, of which the partners in the chat are not always aware, resides in the linguistic resources they employ.

The analysis revealed that the linguistic resources employed by the volunteers were useful in establishing an emotional contact with the help-seeker and in enhancing cognitive changes. The major linguistic characteristic that contributed to the creation of intimacy and trust was the use of unpretentious and familiar language. This type of language was manifested in the high frequency of moderating expressions, conditional sentences, and words retrieved from the semantic field of intimacy. This unpretentious language was helpful in mitigating the effect of inequality between the two sides of the therapeutic encounter by shaping an egalitarian communication that stressed the human similarities between the help-giver and the help-seeker. The value of the human-oriented approach for the effective outcome of psychotherapy was emphasized by the humanistic approach in psychology (Rogers, 1951), which claimed that the "person" rather than the "patient" is the therapist's partner. This approach earned empirical support in a study examining the telephonic interactions between troubled callers and trained volunteers (Gilat & Rosenau, 2011). One of the major characteristics of helpful interactions was the egalitarian relationship between the volunteer and the help-seeker.

The linguistic feature that helped bring about a cognitive change in the effective interactions that were analyzed in the present study is the use of words and expressions with a positive signification. In some cases, the volunteer employed such expressions, and in others, the volunteer highlighted expressions written by the help-seeker and exploited them to suggest a more positive perspective.

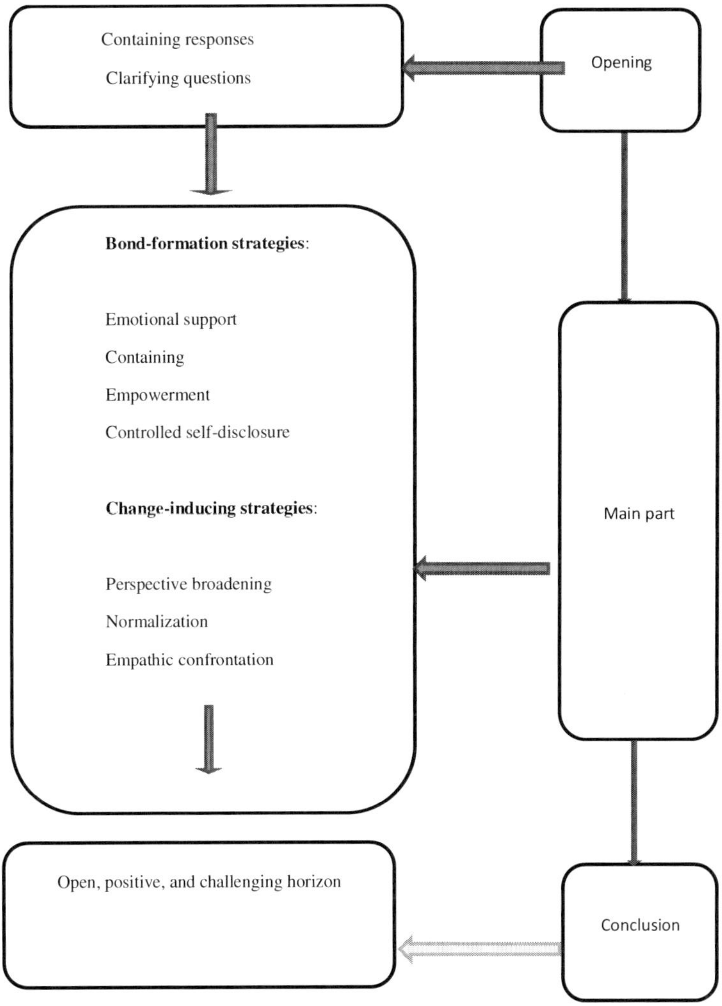

Figure 3. A model of interaction in personal chat.

Structure of the interaction: In most chats, a typical three-part structure could be identified. The first part was the beginning, whose aim was to engender trust, enhance the help-seeker's openness, and expand the discourse by posing clarifying questions. The second part comprised two components that appeared in two steps: creating a supportive environment followed by suggesting that the help-seeker adopt alternative perspectives – less threatening and more encouraging than the perspectives introduced at the beginning of the chat. The third part concluded the encounter and consisted of presenting an open and challenging horizon and sometimes suggesting practical ideas for coping with the problem.

CONCLUSION

Empirical evidence regarding the helpfulness of the emotional first aid rendered by trained volunteers on the Internet is scarce. The first study reported in this chapter revealed that help-seekers perceive this type of assistance as helpful since it increases emotional well-being, induces cognitive change, and suggests practical ways of coping with problems. This evidence supports previous studies regarding the efficacy of trained volunteers in emotional first aid via the telephone helpline, and encourages the use of volunteers as agents of assistance in the field of mental health. Moreover, the evidence not only helps dispel the doubts surrounding the legitimacy of providing psychological assistance via the online environment, but also constitutes a sound basis for expanding the use of this type of service, thereby enabling larger populations to benefit from it.

In the second study reported here, an in-depth, qualitative analysis of transcripts of chats that had been evaluated as helpful was conducted. This analysis revealed the characteristics of helpful interactions that can be converted into a training program for volunteers – as well as professionals – who specialize in rendering psychological assistance on the Internet.

Chapter 8

LIMITATIONS, RISKS, AND ETHICAL DILEMMAS

ABSTRACT

The features of the online environment give rise to conditions that enhance the efficacy of psychological assistance but at the same time pose limitations, create risks, and raise ethical dilemmas that should be considered in order to better exploit the online environment for emotional assistance. These limitations, risks, and ethical dilemmas are presented and discussed in the present chapter. First, we shall put forward limitations and risks that are common to professional therapy and emotional first aid, namely, dependence on technology, faking, lack of non-verbal cues, and encouragement of dangerous behaviors such as suicide and eating disorders. We shall then present ethical dilemmas that are specific to the context of volunteer-based emotional first aid, namely, dealing with recurrent help-seekers as well as with suicidal individuals who contact a service that offers assistance but refuse to cooperate with its efforts to help them deal with their crises.

INTRODUCTION

The idea of administering psychological treatment via the online environment was not welcomed by mental health professionals at the beginning of the Internet era. Many of them opposed the very idea that an emotional relationship can be established via a technologically-mediated environment. They also posited possible risks for both patients and therapists as a result of the characteristics of the online environment. An example of the dissenting voices can be found in a lecture given at the annual meeting of the American Psychological Association (APA) by Holmes, who asserted: "You can't do psychotherapy on the net, yet" (1997).

The opposition to rendering emotional assistance via the Internet was not limited to private therapists, but was also evident in the official stance of the mental health establishment. For instance, the APA did not publish specific ethical guidelines for online therapy until 1997 despite the obvious need for them that stems from the novel context in which the encounter between therapist and client occurs. The American Association of Clinical Social Workers published an explicit statement of opposition to the administering of emotional assistance via the Internet (Rummell & Joyce, 2010).

The opposition to assimilating online therapy within the existing bank of psychotherapy methods and environments can be explained by the phenomenon of resistance to change that characterizes the attitude of individuals and groups toward the implementation of any changes in their environments. However, this opposition can be explained by another factor that is more rational and is related to the limitations and risks resulting from utilizing the online environment for the purpose of psychological assistance. Offering psychological assistance in a technologically-mediated environment requires that both help-givers and clients cope with limitations such as a lack of non-verbal cues and dependence on the technology. Furthermore, it evokes ethical dilemmas such as dealing with suicidal threats from anonymous help-seekers. It is necessary to be aware of these limitations and dilemmas and develop strategies for coping with them in order to better exploit the potential of the online environment for rendering psychological assistance.

Unlike professional therapy, volunteer-based emotional first aid via the Internet was deemed a natural extension of the highly-valued, traditional mental health service, namely, the telephone hotline, and was implemented by organizations providing telephone assistance (Barak, 2007; Gilat & Shahar, 2007; Wilson & Lester, 2002). However, these services had to cope with limitations, risks, and ethical dilemmas from their very inception. While some of the risks and dilemmas are common to professional and para-professional online services that render psychological assistance, others are unique to the emotional first aid provided by trained volunteers. This chapter presents the two types of limitations and dilemmas and describes the strategies that were developed to cope with them.

Dependence on Technology

"The first time we met it was really frustrating because of the technology. We were both there. We were both excited. Not only was it technology but me being not so technologically-advanced either. I think there was one time where the server was down. We had barely started talking and the server shut me out. And another time, I didn't realize I had pressed return like a hundred times and the computer was going wacko" (Haberstroh et al., 2007, p. 274).

This quotation, taken from a study examining the experience of research participants who were engaged in online counseling, exemplifies one of the limitations of providing psychological assistance via the Internet, namely, dependence on technology. Psychological assistance on the Internet always occurs within the online environment and is consequently liable to suffer impairments resulting directly from technological problems or human errors in applying the technology. For instance, a therapeutic encounter via personal chat may come to an abrupt halt due to problems in the computer or a power failure; an email sent by a therapist to her client may arrive at someone else's mailbox due to an incorrect email address. The effect of limitations resulting from technological causes on processes of emotional first aid can be stronger than their effect on professional therapy because most of the clients who seek emotional first aid remain anonymous, and it is impossible to contact them after the unexpected termination of the interaction.

The damage caused by technological problems is limited not only to an interruption in the continuity of the interaction, but may be intensified due to the inevitable interpretation of the breakdown by the partners in the therapeutic encounter. Technological problems almost always occur with one party only. The other is unaware of the real reason underlying the problem and may ascribe a psychological interpretation to it that is liable to sabotage the relationship. For instance, a therapist who is involved in an email-based therapy and fails to receive an email from the client on time may interpret this as a symptom of resistance. This may cause him/her to resume the process on the basis of an erroneous assumption.

The abrupt termination of interactions due to technological problems is more difficult to cope with in emotional first aid because the help-seeker is anonymous and cannot be reached in order to determine the reason for the sudden termination. Our experience in ERAN shows that some volunteers attribute such abrupt endings to their own "human errors" and become frustrated. In one case, a volunteer reported an "error" of this kind at the supervisory session. The very next day, an email from the help-seeker arrived in which the latter apologized for the abrupt termination of their chat, explaining that it had been caused by a power failure. The help-seeker went on to compliment the volunteer on her helpful chat...

Faking

The online environment grants individuals a wish that was possible only in fairytales in the pre-Internet era: the ability to remain unseen and unheard when communicating with others. While this ability can promote the efficacy of psychological assistance by increasing self-disclosure (see Chapter 2), it can also pose an obstacle by allowing help-seekers to select their identity and their narrative, which are not necessarily authentic. In other words, online communication creates convenient conditions for faking.

When clients present false identities, they make it extremely difficult for therapists to meet ethical standards. For instance, an adolescent may fake his/her age in order to avoid the necessity of obtaining parental consent for undergoing therapy; or a therapist may not be certain whether the client who is chatting with him/her in the second session is the same person who chatted in the first one.

In order to cope with the possibility of faking, professional therapists are advised to take measures such as insisting on a face-to-face meeting prior to commencing therapy, or asking the client at the beginning of each session to sum up the previous one or to describe the impact the session had upon him/her (Rummell & Joyce, 2010).

The risk of faking is more difficult to handle in emotional first aid than in professional therapy. The measures that are taken for coping with faking in professional therapy are not applicable in the context of emotional first aid, where maintaining the help-seekers' anonymity is one of the leading principles. ERAN violates the anonymity of help-seekers in emergency situations only, namely, suicidal threats or abuse of youngsters. In no other cases are the identity of the help-seeker and the authenticity of his/her narrative checked. Our experience in ERAN shows that volunteers occasionally doubt the authenticity of the story. These cases evoke an ethical and professional dilemma. On the one hand, manipulation of identity can be viewed as a legitimate behavior in emotional first aid. For instance, adolescents can test their emerging identity by means of an interpersonal interaction with the volunteer in which they adopt a different identity. On the other hand, it is impossible for help-givers to establish an emotional bond with the help-seeker if they doubt the genuineness of the help-seeker's identity. The resolution of this dilemma is left to the discretion of each volunteer when confronted with this challenging situation.

Lack of Non-verbal Communication

The lack of non-verbal cues within the communication that occurs in most channels of the online environment is considered to be the most serious limitation of the Internet as a context for emotional assistance. Eye contact, facial expressions, body movements, prosody, and many other non-verbal means play a major role in psychological diagnosis and in establishing an emotional bond between help-giver and help-seeker. The diagnosis is based not only on the overt information provided by the help-seeker, but also on the hidden parts of the "self" that are vital in order to obtain a comprehensive portrait of his/her condition, and of which the help-seeker is less aware. Non-verbal cues provide access to these hidden parts. As regards the therapeutic process, the lack of non-verbal cues impairs the ability to establish trust and develop a therapeutic alliance. For instance, the manifestation of empathy toward the help-seeker, which constitutes a major component in creating an emotional bond, is achieved via facial expressions and intonation.

Some critics of online therapy claim that non-verbal communication is crucial for the process of psychological assistance (Holmes, 1997). This claim completely negates the legitimacy of providing psychological assistance via the online environment. The response to this criticism is based on empirical evidence regarding the establishment of emotional relationships on the Internet. From the very onset of online therapy, clinical experience and empirical research presented substantial evidence of powerful emotional processes that developed in interpersonal communication on the Internet. (This evidence is presented in detail in Chapters 2 and 4.)

How can the establishment of an emotional bond on the Internet be explained? Text-based communication generates linguistic devices that compensate for the lack of non-verbal cues that are embedded in spoken communication. One type of compensation resides in linguistic resources that transmit extra-linguistic messages. These include, for instance, the frequent use of words from the same semantic field (Gilat & Tobin, 2009), repetitions of words, and the use of metaphors and other figurative forms (Kupferberg & Gilat, 2012). In most cases, the writers are not aware that they are using these means to convey messages. Another type of communication is the use of emoticons (emotional icons), which are pictorial representations of facial expressions such as the smiley ☺.

Encouraging Dangerous Behavior

> "I prefer to talk via the personal chat [rather than face-to-face] because I don't need to lie, you don't have to cope with facial expressions and emotions, and I can be real, disgusting and anti-social, exactly as I like."

This quotation, taken from an online support group, illustrates one of the major features of the communication on the Internet: the lowering of the barriers to openness and to the direct expression of personal feelings, known as the "disinhibition effect" (see Chapter 2). Although this feature enhances the efficacy of psychological assistance by promoting self-disclosure, it also has a potentially negative and even destructive effect on interpersonal communication and on the well-being of the surfers.

One of the domains in which the dangerous aspect of the communication on the Internet is manifested is suicidal behavior. There are websites, in the form of personal blogs, forums, web pages, Facebook, and so on, which encourage people to commit suicide and even suggest ways to do so. These sites are easily accessible by means of search engines. Their contents glorify suicide and portray it as a desirable solution for pain and anguish. They include suicide letters written by individuals who committed suicide, stories about the suicides of famous people, detailed descriptions of ways of committing suicide, and trenchant criticism of mental health assistance that aims to prevent suicide (Baume et al., 1997; Recupero et al., 2008; Westerlund, 2012). These contents may be dangerous for individuals who are in the throes of acute mental pain and view their problems as insurmountable. They experience a severe conflict between the desire to escape the unbearable mental pain by committing suicide and the natural urge to live. Exposure to pro-suicide messages and detailed descriptions of suicides committed by famous personages may reinforce the notion of suicide and motivate them to resolve their inner conflicts in this manner.

The phenomenon of encouraging suicide through exposure to pro-suicide messages on the media is not new, and has been labeled "the Werther Effect". This term was coined in the wake of Johann Wolfgang von Goethe's famous book, *The Sorrows of Young Werther*, which was published in 1774 and was purported to have triggered a wave of suicide events, primarily among youngsters. Researchers assert that exposure to pro-suicide contents on the Internet is more powerful than such exposure via other media since the Internet boasts features such as high accessibility, use of multi-media stimuli, and ease of communication with others (Baume et al., 1997).

Another example of dangerous behavior that is encouraged on the Internet is Anorexia Nervosa (AN). The most dangerous disease in the category of eating disorders, AN is characterized by self-starvation, a sharp decrease in weight, and a distorted body image. It is a disease that can cause death if the patients (mostly adolescents and young women) fail to receive treatment. Unfortunately, two of the characteristics of AN are the eschewal of treatment as a result of denying the problem, and/or harboring a negative attitude toward therapy and therapists (Franko& Rolfe, 1996; Goldner, Birmingham & Smye, 1997). The Internet, which contains websites that encourage anorectic individuals to perpetuate their disorder, may exacerbate their reluctance to receive assistance. These websites are known as "Pro-Ana" and contain personal blogs explaining the advantages of being anorectic, pictures of very thin models, and practical advice for perpetuating the AN.

While it is impossible to prevent the existence of websites that encourage dangerous behaviors, it is both possible and essential to increase the number and the quality of online services offering psychological and instrumental assistance. Volunteer-based emotional first-aid services can play an invaluable role in achieving this objective.

Ethical Dilemmas in Emotional First Aid

Emotional first aid differs from professional therapy in several characteristics that have implications as regards the limitations and ethical dilemmas that arise in the process of providing online assistance: the individuals who seek emotional first aid can remain anonymous; the assistance is offered by trained volunteers who are not professionals in the field of mental health; the volunteers generally remain anonymous vis-à-vis the help-seekers; and the purpose of the assistance is to render emotional support and achieve an immediate improvement in the help-seeker's emotional welfare rather than enduring changes in his/her condition. In addition, emotional first aid is provided in a single-session intervention rather than during the course of an ongoing relationship.

Some of the limitations and ethical dilemmas, such as the dependence on technology and the lack of nonverbal cues presented above, are common to the two types of psychological assistance. Others are specific to the context and the service of emotional first aid, and are presented in the following sections.

One ethical dilemma that specifically concerns emotional first-aid services derives from the phenomenon of recurrent help-seekers. This phenomenon was investigated in the context of emotional first aid via telephone hotline (Lester, Brockopp & Blum, 1973), and the findings revealed that the population of hotline callers can be divided into two groups on the basis of the frequency of seeking assistance. The first group comprises first-time help-seekers and people who contact the agency during a limited period, usually in times of crisis. Individuals in this group usually expect problem-focused assistance.

The second group comprises individuals who contact the agency frequently, sometimes even several times a day, over an extended period – even years. They usually live in an ongoing state of loneliness and require a constant external source of emotional support in order to counterbalance their stressful experiences and enable them to perform their daily routine. Although empirical evidence pertaining to recurrent help-seekers on the Internet is scarce, the experience garnered by ERAN reveals that their characteristics are similar to recurrent help-seekers on the telephone.

The phenomenon of recurrent help-seekers raises a dilemma that is manifested in a conflict between two opposing approaches. One approach asserts that recurrent help-seekers should be given limitless assistance because not only is it vital for maintaining their normal functioning, but they lack alternative sources of assistance. If they are not permitted to receive emotional support whenever they need it, their mental condition may deteriorate and they may require hospitalization.

The other approach states that limitless compliance with the help-seekers' expectations increases their dependence on external sources and prevents them from developing internal coping resources. The assistance offered them should be limited in its frequency (e.g., one chat per day). In addition, full compliance with recurrent help-seekers' appeals for assistance reduces the availability of the service to first-time help-seekers. The recommendation of the above-mentioned authors was not to adopt either approach exclusively, but rather to decide upon the appropriate one for every help-seeker.

Another ethical dilemma arises in interactions with individuals who talk about committing suicide. If the help-seeker rejects the efforts of the volunteer to change his/her suicidal intention, and the volunteer evaluates the risk as high, emergency forces are dispatched in order to locate the help-seeker and save his/her life. The intervention is carried out contrary to the help-seeker's explicit wishes. This situation evokes an ethical dilemma which is manifested in a conflict between two major principles that are embedded in the ethical code of ERAN and many other emotional first-aid services, namely, respecting help-seeker's anonymity on the one hand and saving a life on the other. Volunteers are not expected to resolve this dilemma each time they face it during an interaction with a suicidal individual. They are instructed to act according to the ethical code developed by the agency. Although most of the volunteer-based organizations deem forced intervention for saving a life a legitimate decision, some organizations consider anonymity to be paramount and do not dispatch emergency forces if the help-seeker declines to provide identifying details (Bongar, 1991).

CONCLUSION

Limitations, risks, and ethical dilemmas are inevitable when psychological assistance is provided on the Internet. Help-givers – both professional therapists and trained volunteers – should be aware of them in order to increase their efficacy as online counselors. They should also be acquainted with the strategies that have been developed in order to cope with these obstacles and learn how to apply such strategies in their practice. This knowledge should be imparted in the training process for online counselors and in supervisory sessions. Ethical dilemmas should also be discussed by experts in the fields of professional therapy, emotional first aid, and ethics. While such discussions would not produce absolute solutions to the dilemmas, they could generate guidelines for coping with them that would be incorporated in the ethical codes for providing psychological assistance.

References

Adis, M. E. & Mahalik, J. R. (2003). Men, masculinity and contexts of help-seeking. *American Psychologist*, *58*, 5-14.

Alonzo, M. & Aiken, M. (2004). Flaming in electronic communication. *Decision Support Systems*, *36*, 205-213.

Barak, A. (2007). Emotional support and suicide prevention through the Internet: A field project study. *Computers in Human Behavior, 23*, 971-984.

Barak, A., Boniel-Nissim, M. & Suler, J. (2008). Fostering empowerment in online support groups. *Computers in Human Behavior*, *24*, 1867-1883.

Bareket-Bojmel, B. & Shahar, G. (2011). Emotional and interpersonal consequences of self-disclosure in a lived, online interaction. *Journal of Social and Clinical Psychology*, *30*,732-759.

Bauer, S., Wolf, M., Haug, S. & Kordy, H. (2011). The effectiveness of internet chat groups in relapse prevention after inpatient psychotherapy. *Psychotherapy Research*, *21*, 219-226.

Baume, P., Cantor, C. H. & Rolfe, A. (1997). Cybersuicide: The role of interactive suicide notes on the internet. *Crisis*, *18*, 73-79.

Becker, K., Mayer, M., Nagenborg, M., El-Faddagh, N. & Schmidt, M. H. (2004). Parasuicide online: Can suicide websites trigger suicidal behavior in predisposed adolescents? *Nordic Journal of Psychiatry*, *58*, 111-114.

Bongar, B. (1991). *The suicidal patient: Clinical and legal standards of care.* Washington DC: American Psychological Association.

Boniel-Nissim, M. & Barak, A. (2011). The therapeutic value of adolescents' blogging about social-emotional difficulties. *Psychological Services*. Advance online publication. doi: 10.1037/a0026664.

Bowlby, J. (1969). *Attachment and loss. Volume 1: Attachment.* New York, NY: Basic Books.

Brockopp, G. W. (1973). An emergency telephone service: The development of a presence. In D. Lester & G. W. Brockopp (Eds.), *Crisis intervention and counseling by telephone* (pp. 9-23). Springfield, IL: Charles C. Thomas.

Buchanan, H. & Coulson, N. S. (2007). Accessing dental anxiety in online support groups: An exploratory qualitative study of motives and experiences. *Patient Education and Counseling*, *66*, 263-269.

Campbell, R., Wasco, S. M., Ahrens, C. E., Sefl, T. & Barnes, H. E. (2001). Preventing the "second rape": Rape survivors' experiences with community service providers. *Journal of Interpersonal Violence*, *16*, 1239-1259.

Caplan, G. (1964). *Principles of preventive psychiatry*. New York, NY: Basic Books.

Caplan, G. (1974). *Support systems and community mental health*. New York, NY: Behavioral Publications.

Chen, S., Jordan, C. & Thompson, S. (2006). The effect of cognitive behavioral therapy (CBT) on depression: The role of problem-solving appraisal. *Research on Social Work Practice*, *16*, 500-510.

Chester, A. & Glass, C. A. (2006). Online counseling: A descriptive analysis of therapy services on the Internet. *British Journal of Guidance & Counselling*, *34*, 145-160.

Cialdini, R. B. (2003). Crafting normative messages to protect the environment. *Current Directions in Psychological Research*, *12*, 105-109.

Clark, D. C. & Fawcett, J. (1992). Review of empirical risk factors for evaluation of the suicidal patient. In B. Bongar (Ed.), *Suicide: Guidelines for assessment, management and treatment*. New York, NY: Oxford University Press.

Cohen, S. & Wills, T. A. (1985). Stress, social support and buffering hypothesis. *Psychological Bulletin*, *98*, 10-57.

Cook, J. E. & Doyle, C. (2002). Working alliance in online therapy as compared to face-to-face therapy: Preliminary results. *Cyber Psychology & Behavior*, *5*, 95-105.

Coyne, J. C. (1976). Depression and the response of others. *Journal of Abnormal Psychology*, *85*, 186-193.

Crystal, D. (2000). *Language and the Internet*. Cambridge, UK: Cambridge University Press.

Etzersdorfer, E., Sonneck, G. & Nagel-Kuess, S. (1992). Newspaper reports and suicide. *The New England Journal of Medicine*, *38*, 453-457.

Fink, J. & Colon, Y. (1999). Digital digging: Group therapy online. In J. Fink (Ed.), *How to use computers and cyberspace in the clinical practice of psychotherapy* (pp. 65-81). Northvaic, NJ: Jason Aronson.

Fowler, D. E. & McGee, R. K. (1973). Assessing the performance of telephone crisis workers: The development of a technical effectiveness scale. In D. Lester & G. W. Brockopp (Eds.), *Crisis intervention and counseling by telephone* (pp. 277-286). Springfield, IL: Charles C. Thomas.

Franko, D. L. & Rolfe, S. (1996). Countertransference in the treatment of patients with eating disorders. *Psychiatry*, 108-115.

Freud, S. (1959). Analysis of a phobia in a five-year-old boy. *Collected Papers*. New York, NY: Basic Books.

Fukkink, R. & Hermanns, J. (2009). Counseling children at a helpline: Chatting or calling? *Journal of Community Psychology*, *37*(8), 939-948.

Garland, A. F. & Zigler, E. F. (1994). Psychological correlates of help-seeking attitudes among children and adolescents. *American Journal of Orthopsychiatry*, *64*, 586-593.

Gilat, I. (2008). *Supportive response to suicidal messages in an online support group: An action-theory approach.* Dissertation submitted to Ben-Gurion University of the Negev, Beer Sheba, Israel.

Gilat, I. (2010) *Characteristics of calls for emotional first aid in 2009.* A research Report. The Israeli Association of Emotional First Aid.

Gilat, I., Ezer, H. & Sagee, R. (2010). Help-seeking attitudes among Arab and Jewish adolescents in Israel. *British Journal of Guidance and Counselling*, *38*(2), 205-218.

Gilat, I., Ezer, H. & Sagee, R. (2011). Seeking help by adolescents from traditional and online sources. *Megamot, 57, 616 – 640* (Hebrew)

Gilat, I. & Latzer, Y. (2007). Characteristics of calls to the Israeli hotline during the Intifada. *Community Mental Health Journal*, *43*, 401-420.

Gilat, I., Lobel, T. & Gil, T. E. (1998). Characteristics of calls to the Israeli hot lines during the Gulf War. *American Journal of Community Psychology*, *26*, 697-704.

Gilat, I. & Reshef, E. (in press). The perceived helpfulness of rendering emotional first aid via email. *British Journal of Guidance and Counselling.*

Gilat, I. & Rosenau, S. (2004). How to be released from the jaws of death: Analysis of an online suicidal conversation with an adolescent boy. *Social Educational Work*, *20*, 61-84. (Hebrew)

Gilat, I. & Rosenau, S. (2011). Volunteers' perspective of effective interactions with hotline callers: Qualitative study. *British Journal of Guidance and Counselling*, 39, 325-337.

Gilat, I. & Shahar, G. (2007). Emotional first aid for a suicide crisis: Comparison between telephonic hotline and Internet. *Psychiatry: Interpersonal and Biological Processes*, *70*, 12-18.

Gilat, I. & Shahar, G. (2009). Suicide prevention by online support groups: An Action Theory-based model of emotional first aid. *Archives of Suicide Research*, *13*, 52-63.

Gilat, I. & Tobin, Y. (2009). "I am so tired of this life": A semiotic analysis of suicidal messages on the Internet. In L. Sher & A. Vilens (Eds.), *Internet and Suicide* (pp. 169-184). New York, NY: Nova Science Publishers.

Gilat, I., Tobin, Y. & Shahar, G. (2011). Offering support to suicidal participants in an online support group. *Archives of Suicide Research, 15*,195-206.

Goldner, E. M., Birmingham, C. L. & Smye, V. (1997). Addressing treatment refusal in anorexia nervosa: Clinical, ethical and legal issues. In D. M. Garner & P. E. Garfinkel (Eds.), *Handbook of treatment for eating disorders* (pp. 450-461). New York, NY: Guilford Press.

Gould, M. S., Greenberg, T., Velting, D. M. & Shaffer, D. (2003). Youth suicide risk and preventive interventions: A review of the past ten years. *Journal of the American Academy of Child and Adolescent Psychiatry*, *42*, 386-405.

Gould, M. S., Munfakh, J. L. H., Lubell, K., Klienman, M. & Parker, S. (2002). Seeking help from the internet during adolescence. *Journal of the American Academy of Child and Adolescent Psychiatry*, *41*, 1182-1190.

Grunbaum, J. A., Kann, L. & Kinchen, S. A. (2002). *Youth risk behavior surveillance United States, 2001*. MMWR CDC SurveillSumm 51 (SS4), 1-64.

Gulec, H., Moessner, M., Mezei, A., Kohls, E., Tury, F. & Bauer, S. (2011). Internet-based maintenance treatment for patients with eating disorders. *Professional Psychology: Research and Practice*, *42*, 479-486.

Haberstroh, S., Duffey, T., Evans, M., Gee, R. & Trepal, H. (2007).The experience of on-line counseling. *Journal of Mental Health Counseling*, *29*, 269-282.

Heilig, S. M., Farberow, N. L., Litman, R. E. & Shneidman, E. S. (1968). The role of nonprofessional volunteers in a suicide prevention center. *Community Mental Health Journal*, *4*, 267-295.

Hollander, E. M. (2001). Cyber community in the valley of the shadow of death. *Journal of Loss and Trauma*, *6*, 135-146.

Holmes, L. G. (1997). *You can't do psychotherapy on the net, yet*. Paper presented at the annual meeting of the American Psychological Association, Chicago, IL.

Horvath, A. O. & Luborsky, L. (1993).The role of the therapeutic alliance in psychotherapy. *Journal of Consulting and Clinical Psychology*, *61*, 561-573.

Houston, T. K., Cooper, L. A. & Ford, D. E. (2002). Internet support groups for depression: A 1-year prospective cohort study. *The American Journal of Psychiatry*, *159*(12), 2062-2068.

Isometsa, E. T., Aro, H. M., Henriksson, M. M., Heikkinen, M. E. & Lonnquist, J. K. (1994). Suicide in major depression in different treatment settings. *Journal of Clinical Psychiatry*, *55*, 523-527.

Joiner, T. E. (1995). The price of soliciting and receiving negative feedback: Self-verification theory as a vulnerability to depression theory. *Journal of Abnormal Psychology*, *104*, 364-372.

Joiner, T. E. (2005). *Why people die by suicide*. Cambridge, MA: Harvard University Press.

Joiner, T. E., Pettit, J. W., Walker, R. L., Voelz, Z. R., Cruz, J., Rudd, M. D. & Lester, D. (2002). Perceived burdensomeness and suicidality: Two studies on the suicide notes of those attempting and those completing suicide. *Journal of Social and Clinical Psychology*, *21*, 531-545.

Kazdin, A. E. & Blasé, S. L. (2011). Rebooting psychotherapy research and practice to reduce the burden of mental illness. *Perspectives on Psychological Science*, *6*, 21-37.

King, R., Bambling, M., Lloyd, C., Gomurra, R., Smith, S., Reid, W. & Wegner, K. (2006). Online counseling: The motives and experiences of young people who choose the internet instead of face to face or telephone counseling. *Counseling and Psychotherapy Research*, *6*, 169-174.

Kupferberg, I. & Gilat, I. (2012).The discursive self-construction of suicidal help seekers in computer-mediated discourse. *Communication & Medicine*, *9*, 23-35.

Lange, A., Rietdijk, D., Hudcovicova, M., van de Ven, J., Schrieken, B. & Emmelkamp, P. M. G. (2003). Interpay: A controlled randomized trial of the standardized treatment of posttraumatic stress through the internet. *Journal of Consulting & Clinical Psychology*, *71*, 901-909.

Larson, R. & Ham, M. (1993). Stress and "storm and stress" in early adolescence: The relationship of negative events with dysphoric affect. *Developmental Psychology*, *29*,130-140.

Latzer, Y. & Gilat, I. (2000). Calls to the Israeli hotline from individuals who suffer from eating disorders: An epidemiological study. *Eating Disorders*, *8*, 31-42.

Lazar, A. & Erera, I. (1998). Telephone helplines as social support. *International Social Work*, *14*, 89-101.

Lazarus, R. S. & Folkman, S. (1984). *Stress, appraisal and coping*. New York, NY: Springer.

Lebow, J. (1998). Not just talk, maybe some risk: The therapeutic potentials and pitfalls of computer-mediated conversation. *Journal of Marital and Family Therapy*, *24*, 203-206.

Leibert, T., Archer, J., Munson, J. & York, G. (2006). An exploratory study of client perception of internet counseling and the alliance. *Journal of Mental Health Counseling*, *28*, 69-83.

Lester, D. (1997). The effectiveness of suicide prevention centers: A review. *Suicide and Life Threatening Behavior*, *27*, 304-31.

Lester, D. (2008-2009). The use of the Internet for counseling the suicidal individual: Possibilities and drawbacks. *Omega*, *58*, 233-250.

Lester, D. (2009). The use of the Internet for counseling the suicidal individual: Possibilities and drawbacks. *Omega*, *58*(3), 233-250.

Lester, D., Brockopp, G. W. & Blum, D. (1973).The chronic caller. In D. Lester & G. W. Brockopp (Eds.), *Crisis intervention and counseling by telephone* (pp. 175-192). Springfield, IL: Charles C. Thomas.

Martin, D. J., Garske, J. P. & Davis, M. K. (2000). Relation of the therapeutic alliance with outcome and other variables: A meta-analytic review. *Journal of Consulting and Clinical Psychology*, *68*, 438-450.

McGee, R. K. & Jennings, B. (2002). Ascending to "lower levels": The case for nonprofessional crisis workers. In D. Lester & G. W. Brockopp (Eds.), *Crisis intervention and counseling by telephone* (pp. 231-241). Springfield, IL: Charles C. Thomas.

McLuhan, M. (1964). *Understanding media: The extensions of man.* New York, NY: Signet.

Miller, J. K. & Gergen, J. G. (1998). Life on the line: The therapeutic potentials of computer-mediated conversation. *Journal of Marital and Family Therapy*, *24*, 2, 189-203.

Mishara, B. L., Changon, F., Diagle, M., Balan, B., Raymond, S., Marcoux, I., Bardon, C., Campbell, J. & Berman, E. (2007). Comparing models of helper behavior to actual practice in telephone crisis intervention: A silent monitoring study of calls to the U.S. 1-800-SUICIDE network. *Suicide and Life Threatening Behavior*, *37*, 291-307.

Motto, J. A., Brooks, R. M., Ross, C. P. & Allen, N. H. (1974). *Standards for suicide prevention and crisis centers.* New York, NY: Behavioral Publications.

Offer, D., Howard, H. I., Schonert, K. A. & Ostrov, E. (1991). To whom do adolescents turn for help? Differences between disturbed and non-disturbed adolescents. *Journal of the American Academy of Child and Adolescent Psychiatry*, *30*, 623-630.

Parks, M. R. & Roberts, L. D. (1998). "Making MOOsic": The development of personal relationships online and a comparison to their off-line counterparts. *Journal of Social and Personal Relationships*, *15*, 517-537.

Patterson, D., Greeson, M. & Campbell, R. (2009). Understanding rape survivors' decisions not to seek help from formal social systems. *Health & Social Work*, *14*,127-136.

Pennebaker, J. W. (1997). Writing about emotional experiences as a therapeutic process. *Psychological Science*, *8*, 162-166.

Pennebaker, J. W., Mehl, M. R. & Niederhoffer, K. G. (2003). Psychological aspects of natural language use: Our words, our selves. *Annual Review of Psychology*, *54*, 547-577.

Phillips, D. (1974). The influence of suggestion on suicide: Substantial and theoretical implications of the Werther Effect. *American Sociology Review*, *39*, 340-354.

Powell, T. (1998). Online counseling: A profile and descriptive analysis. Available at: www.netpsych.com/Powell.htm (22 July, 2003).

Raviv, A., Sills, R., Raviv, A. & Wilensky, P. (2000). Adolescents' help-seeking behavior: The difference between self- and other-referral. *Journal of Adolescence, 23*, 721-740.

Recupero, P. R., Harms, S. E. & Noble, J. M. (2008). Googling suicide: Surfing for suicide information on the internet. *Journal of Clinical Psychiatry, 69*, 878-888.

Reese, R. J., Collie, W. C. & Brossart, D. F. (2002). Effectiveness of telephone counseling: A field-based investigation. *Journal of Counseling Psychology, 49*, 233-242.

Rogers, C. (1951). *Client-centered therapy*. Boston, MA: Houghton Mifflin.

Rogers, C. (1980). *A way of being*. Boston, MA: Houghton Mifflin.

Rosenau, S. & Gilat, I. (2011). "My life is breaking into pieces" – Distress of adolescents as reflected in emails. In H. Ezer, I. Gilat & R. Sagee (Eds.), *"I am all alone in this story" – Young people in Israel cope with stressful situations* (pp. 41-83). Tel Aviv: The MOFET Institute. (Hebrew)

Roy, H. & Gillett, T. (2008). E-mail: A new technique for forming a therapeutic alliance with high-risk young people failing to engage with mental health services? A case study. *Clinical Child Psychology and Psychiatry, 13*, 95-103.

Rubin, Z. (1975). Disclosing oneself to a stranger: Reciprocity and its limits. *Journal of Experimental Social Psychology, 11*, 233-260.

Rummell, C. M. & Joyce, N. R. (2010). "So what do u want to work on 2day?": The ethical implications of online counseling. *Ethics and Behavior, 20*, 482-496.

Sarason, I., Sarason, B. & Pierce, G. (1990). Relationship-specific social support: Toward a model for analysis of supportive interactions. In B. Burlson, T. Albrecht & I. Sarason (Eds.), *Communication of social support: Messages, interactions, relationships and community* (pp. 91-112). Thousand Oaks, CA: Sage.

Shneidman, E. (1996). *The suicidal mind*. New York, NY: Oxford University Press.

Skinner, A. & Zack, J. S. (2004). Counseling and the Internet. *The American Behavioral Scientist, 48*, 434-446.

Stellrecht, N. E., Joiner, T. E. & Rudd, M. D. (2006). Responding to and treating negative interpersonal processes in suicidal depression. *Journal of Clinical Psychology, 62*, 1129-1140.

Stoney, G. (1998). Suicide prevention on the internet. In R. J. Kosky & H. S. Eshkevari (Eds.), *Suicide prevention: The global context* (pp. 237-244). New York, NY: Plenum.

Strauss, A. & Corbin, J. (1990). *Basics of qualitative research: Grounded theory procedures and techniques*. London, UK: Sage Publications.

Suler, J. (2004). The online disinhibition effect. *Cyber Psychology & Behavior*, *7*, 321-326.

Tilov, N., Dear, B. F., Schwencke, G., Andrew, G., Johnston, L., Craske, M. G. & McEvoy, P. (2011).Transdiagnostic internet treatment for anxiety and depression: A randomized controlled trial. *Behavior, Research and Therapy*, *49*, 441-452.

Tishby, M., Turel, M., Gumpel, O., Pinus, U., Ben Lavy, S., Winokour, M. & Szanajderman, S. (2001). Help-seeking attitudes among Israeli adolescents. *Adolescence*, *36*, 249-264.

Trowell, I. (1979). Telephone services. In D. Hankoff & B. Ensidler (Eds.), *Suicide theory and clinical aspects* (pp. 400-409). Littletown, MA: PSG.

Ullman, S. E. &Filipas, H. H. (2001). Correlates of formal and informal support seeking in sexual assault victims. *Journal of Interpersonal Violence*, *16*,1028-1047.

Watson, R. J., McDonald, J. & Pearce, D. C. (2006). An exploration of national calls to Lifeline Australia: Social support or urgent intervention? *British Journal of Guidance and Counselling*, *34*, 471-482.

Weinberg, N., Uken, J. S., Schmale, J. & Adamek, M. (1995). Therapeutic factors: Their presence in a computer-mediated support group. *Social Work with Groups*, *18*, 57-69.

Westerlund, M. (2012).The production of pro-suicide content on the internet: A counter-discourse activity. *New Media & Society, 14,764-780.*

Williams, T. & Douds, J. (1973).The unique contribution of telephone therapy. In D. Lester & G. W. Brockopp (Eds.), *Crisis intervention and counseling by telephone* (pp. 80-88). Springfield, IL: Charles C. Thomas.

Wilson, G. & Lester, D. (2002). Crisis intervention by e-mail. In D. Lester & G. W. Brockopp (Eds.), *Crisis intervention and counseling by telephone* (pp. 212-219). Springfield, IL: Charles C. Thomas.

Wortham, S. (2004). From good student to outcast: Emergence of a classroom identity. *Ethos*, *32*, 164-187.

Yalom, I. D. (1970). *The theory and practice of group psychotherapy*. New York, NY: Basic Books, Inc.

Young, K. S. (2005). An empirical examination of client attitudes towards online counseling. *Cyber Psychology & Behavior*, *8*, 172-177.

INDEX

E

F

K

L

M

N

O

P

Q

R

S

T

U

V

W

Y